MEDICAL ETHICS

A PHYSICIAN'S GUIDE TO CLINICAL MEDICINE

Topic: An Analytical Study to Investigate the Ethical and
Moral Approaches of Physicians in Medical Practices,
Clinical Medicine, and the Physician-Patient Relationship

Emmanuel Adu Addai

Fulton Books, Inc.
Meadville, PA

Published by Fulton Books 2021

ISBN 978-1-64654-954-2 (paperback)
ISBN 978-1-64654-955-9 (digital)

Printed in the United States of America

This Book is dedicated to my beloved deceased:

a. Mary Asantewaa
b. Agartha Animah
c. Margarette Frimpong
d. Aunt Serwaah

CONTENTS

ACKNOWLEDGEMENT

I express my heartfelt gratitude to those people who helped me to complete this project.

First of all, I would like to profusely thank Professors Kayhan Parsi, Nanette Elster and Lena Hatchett who played an invaluable role in my doctoral program in Loyola University Chicago.

I also thank Dr. Amy Van Dyke, who supervised my practicum and my activities for over 6 months. Her guidance was valuable for me during this period. She used to respond to my doubts and queries immediately. I also gained her valuable feedback from time to time.

I am also thankful to Mrs. Gloria Cacara, who helped me in finding literature by providing me information related to the books and database and also taking time to read through the work for me.

My special thanks to the doctors of the two local hospitals, who spent time for me and discussed several cases during their medical practices. They gave me their precious time to talk to me, and they were very friendly and curious about my research.

I am also thankful to the respondents (patients and their relatives). Regardless of their difficult situation, they spent their valuable time in participating the survey.

Great thanks go to my archbishop, Justice Gabriel Yaw Anokye, for giving me the opportunity to study up to this level. I cannot thank him enough. Another thanks go to Emeritus Archbishop of Kumasi, Peter Kwasi Sarpong for his love and support.

I cannot overlook the assistance and great contribution the Ghanaian Catholic Community of St. Anthony, Columbus, Ohio, have made in my education. I am so thankful to them.

I thank my friends and colleagues, especially Frs. Isaac Agbenohevi and Dominic Afrifa Yamoah, for their suggestions and encouragement. Also to all my classmates both in Ghana and United States.

ABSTRACT

Introduction: The medical profession is highly visible and account-able to the public. The value of ethics and morality in this field is immense. Ethics are the codes designed by external entities to control unethical practices in the health-care sector, whereas *morality* is the conscience of the medical practitioners. With the use of both ethics and morality, doctors can successfully handle ethical challenges and dilemmas. However, still some unethical practices have been found in the medical profession. When unethical and unworthy practices come into play, the doctor-patient relationship is likely to be affected.

Objectives: The present dissertation aims to investigate the ethi-cal and moral approaches of the doctors and their impact on patients' health and the relationship between doctors and their patients. With these intentions, we studied the concept of ethics and its significance in clinical settings. The history of medical ethics was also reviewed.

Methods: We used a mixed method of quantitative and qualita-tive analysis with data collected from primary and secondary sources. To explore the ethics and ethical challenges in medical profession, we first reviewed the previous studies. We conducted a qualitative analy-sis of a series of case studies. A total of five cases were analyzed. Along with the qualitative case study analysis, we conducted a survey and a quantitative analysis. For the survey, 110 respondents completed a survey questionnaire.

Results: The results demonstrate the significance of key ethical principles. We found different situations of ethical challenges and dilemmas. We began to understand how doctors can make ethical decisions while still maintaining good relationship with their patients. We found that sometimes doctors have to compromise some ethical principles when presented with complex medical/social situations. The virtues of the doctors were also investigated.

Conclusion: We concluded that even though it may not be possible to follow every ethical principle, doctors should always follow their conscience. It is imperative for them to inculcate values and virtues to serve their patients better and win their trust.

CHAPTER 1

Introduction

1.1. Overview

Ethics and moralities are at the core of human civilizations. *Morals* are the individual principles or one's conscience, while *ethics* are the rules and regulations provided by external sources. Ethical practices in the medical profession are of utmost importance. In fact, this profession needs to be more ethical than any other profession as it is directly related to the patients' health and their lives. Ethical issues are directly associated with life and death. The ethical practices of the medical profession are also known as "clinical ethics," and their goal is to improve the quality of patient care. It is the ethical obligation in medical practices to be competent and to have respect for the patients and their health decisions and maintaining the primacy of the patient's need even under political, economic, and social pressure (Nandi 2000). Trust and respect are two essential principles needed to maintain a good relationship between the doctor and the patient. It is the ethical obligation of medical practitioners to recognize their responsibilities toward the patients and society. According to the principles of medical ethics, the doctor should be dedicated to delivering excellent medical service. In the context of the medical ethics, Beauchamp and Childress (2001) have presented four fundamental principles of medical ethics: (1) respect for autonomy, (2) beneficence, (3) nonmaleficence, and (4) justice. In respect to autonomy, the medical practitioner is expected to respect the right of the patient to accept or refuse any treatment. Beneficence refers to the doctor's duty to act in the best interest of the patient. Nonmaleficence means to not harm the patient, while justice refers to the equal and fair treatment of every patient regardless of his/her social, economic, and political status. These four principles of medical ethics are the pillars of medical ethics on which the edifice of the medical profession rests. Apart from these four principles, Pierre (2014) adds honesty and dignity as two additional principles of medical ethics (see fig. 1).

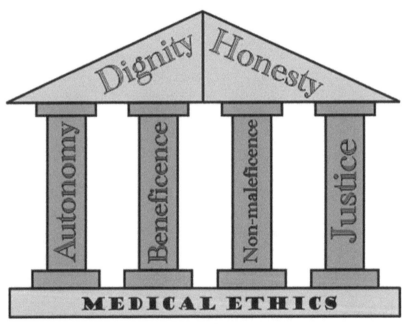

Fig. 1. Bajaj (2014)

The doctor-patient relationship is the foundation of medical ethics. A healthy relationship between the patient and doctor has considerable healing power. That is why the doctor cannot achieve success by just using his clinical knowledge, proficiency, and the technical skills, but rather it depends upon this healthy interpersonal relationship (Raina et al. 2014).

Many times, while dealing with patients and difficult situations, the medical practitioners have to confront moral and ethical dilemmas. Sometimes, the respect for autonomy has to be compromised for the sake of beneficence. At times, the physician's ethics can conflict with the social, economic, and cultural norms. These dilemmas often occur in major issues such as abortion, contraception, euthanasia, confidentiality, truth telling, maintaining relations with patients' relatives, religious issues, traditional medicines, etc. Making decisions in these situations is extremely difficult as the consequences of decision-making are uncertain.

The present thesis attempts to gain a thorough understanding of ethical and moral issues in medical practices. The research has been carried out through case studies, which are based on the ethics in medicine, ethical dilemmas, and the doctor-patient relationship and its impact on ethical practices.

1.2. Research Background and Significance

The proper education related to the practice of medical ethics is an extremely important topic. But this topic has not been taken seriously in medical education, especially in the non-Western countries (Takala 2001). From some years, the topic of medical ethics has been included in medical education as a core domain. However, the application is not adequate. As a result, medical practices are likely to be affected and can sometimes lead to the medical professionals having to respond to legal suits. Hence, there is an acute need of improvement in the study and understanding of medical ethics.

A study was conducted using doctors in Canada researching ethical practices in the medical field. About 52% of the Canadian physicians revealed that they did not have any formal education on medical ethics. About 57% said that they would seek help from the ethics committee if any ethical issues arise (Beauchamp 1998). A similar study was conducted by Yousef et al. (2017) in some Asian countries. In their cross-sectional comparative survey, they attempted to assess the knowledge of the doctors regarding medical ethics. The study observed that the medical practitioners have a strong theoretical knowledge, but they lack knowledge in the actual application of ethical practices in their day-to-day performance of medical duties. In another recent study, those findings were confirmed. Medical students receive theoretical training in medical school, but the training does not address the practical ethical dilemma that is confronted by the doctors while actually practicing (AbuAbah et al. 2019). Doctors are also not aware of several ethical policies such as organ donation regulations, withholding mechanical ventilation, managing conflicts with family members, or seeking advice from the ethics committee (AbuAbah et al. 2019). This shows that the issues related to ethics are faced by the doctors all over the world. That is why the researcher of this thesis perceives it to be crucial to study the common ethical issues in the health-care industry, including the lack of adequate knowledge and the actual implementation of ethics principles.

Inadequate knowledge of medical issues and any number of other such reasons has resulted in growing unethical practices in the medical profession. This tend to likely exist because ethics may have been taught in medical colleges, but these concepts might not have been inculcated in the students. Many unethical practices have been observed by the medical students during their training. There was a survey conducted that involved participation of medical students in their first and fourth years. About 35% of first-year students and 90% of fourth-year students reported observing unethical practices (Satterwhite, Satterwhite, and Enarson 1998). In a recent study with medical students from Malaysia, it was observed that the students had very little or no knowledge about the ethical practices in their profession. In the same study, it was noticed that 75% of the participants had never heard about the Code of Professional Conduct by the Malaysian Medical Council, and 78% of the students were not aware of the Code of Ethics by the Malaysian Medical Association (Yadav et al. 2019).

Medical ethics are directly and indirectly associated with the laws of the respective countries. Doctors should be aware of such laws. The laws regarding medical ethics vary from country to country as they depend upon cultural, social, and political issues. For example, prenatal testing or testing to determine the gender of the fetus is illegal in India. Therefore, it is not an ethical practice to inform the parents of the sex of the fetus prior to its birth. But it is not unethical or illegal if this same practice is conducted in the United Kingdom (UK) or other European countries. This indicates that sometimes the perception of medical ethics is circumstantial. In some cases, the laws are likely to conflict with the ethical practices. In such cases, the physicians are required to disobey the laws that demand unethical behavior. There are several examples of issues that create a great dilemma in the medical profession. That is why there needs to be a larger focus on medical ethics and extensive studies to be undertaken in this area.

1.3. Associating Medical Profession and Ethics

Previous scholars have discussed and debated ethical practices and how they have changed over the course of time (e.g., see Evan [2016] and Saniotis [2007]). However, as mentioned above, their actual practice or implementation is yet to be improved.

Strict adherence to ethical and moral practices is the key to success in the medical profession and subsequently minimize fraud, abuse, and other unethical practices that have become part of this profession. This can only take place with the inculcation of ethical and moral principles among the medical practitioners from the inception of their medical education. The basis of the physicians' professional ethos is associated with what is called the "internal morality" of medical practices. Various medical duties of the practitioners are associated with ethics and the medical profession, such as scientific excellence, commitment to the patients' autonomy, and public accountability (Salloch 2016). This relationship needs to be explored in depth.

1.4. Research Aim and Objectives

Aims	• To investigate the ethical and moral approach of the doctors/physicians in medical practices • To analyze doctor-patient relationship on ethical and moral grounds
Objectives	• To discuss the term ethics • To study the history and background of medical ethics • To analyze case studies on ethical practices • To investigate ethical challenges and dilemmas • To analyze various theories and models of ethics in the context of health care • To shed light on the emergence of hospital committees in the United States • To analyze the changing concept of ethics in modern age

1.5. Research Questions

- What are ethics and their significance in medical professional?
- When can an ethical dilemma take place, and how can the medical professionals face dilemmas while keeping a healthy relationship with their patients?
- When do ethical principles conflict with laws?
- How does ethical decision-making take place during the ethical dilemmas?

To address the research questions, this thesis tries to analyze the existing theories and models of ethics. It will also be crucial to shed light on the historical background of the ethical principles of medical practitioners. There will also be a discussion of what doctors should avoid in order to be considered virtuous and ethical professionals under the current ethical framework.

To address ethical dilemma, the researcher intends to analyze cases in which medical practitioners have to face dilemmas and what the chances are of hampering their relationship with their patients.

In short, the present research intends to shed light on issues related to ethics and moral devices of clinical medicine.

1.6. Scope of the Research

The thesis is singularly focused on ethics and morality in medical practitioners and doctors. The other technical aspects of medical science do not come within the scope of the present study. The scope of the ethics concept is broad; therefore, the research will study different subtopics such as the history of medicine and bioethics, ethical theories and models, the virtues and duties of the medical practitioner, the relationship between the patient and the physician, and ethical issues in medical technology, dealing with difficult patients and their family members and things that the physician should avoid to be virtuous and ethical. The researcher intends to consider the history as well as the modern perspectives of the medical ethics.

Ethical practice is crucial in every sector of business including homeland security, banking, insurance, nursing, military, etc. However, the scope of the present thesis is limited to ethical practices in health care. The research focuses on physicians and does not take into consideration the ethical practice of nurses. Though some of the ethical practices are similar between nurses and doctors, other ethical practices are exclusively related to doctors. The researcher has considered ethical issues in the context of the physician or medical practitioner only.

1.7. Problem Complexity

Globalization and the advancement in information and technology contribute great change in every sector. The health-care sector is no exception. These changes will impact the ethical and moral values as well. New ethical norms have emerged due to technological advancements. This change has a direct impact on doctors, patients, and the entire health-care staff. Considering the wide influence of existing and emerging ethical issues, careful study needs to be undertaken to address them properly.

Today's ethical issues and their complexity require that new ideas and solutions be implemented to address the issues and dilemmas with the ultimate end of improving patients' trust in the medical professionals and doctors.

1.8. Thesis Structure or Outline

This research paper is written in different chapters. The individual chapters are organized in the following way:

Chapter 1: Introduction—The chapter starts with an overview of the scope of the research. Then, the research background and the significance of research are discussed. An association between the medical profession and ethics is described. The researcher then explains the aims and the objectives of the research. Based on the aim, the objectives, and the topic, two research questions have been formulated, and the researcher discusses the scope of the research.

Chapter 2: Literature Review—In this chapter, the researcher has undertaken a review of previous relevant studies on ethics in the medical profession. While reviewing and studying previous literature, careful consideration has been given to the aims, objectives, and research questions addressed in the studies. They provide a roadmap toward exploring relevant information. Following the literature review is a summary of findings. A summary table is provided that incorporates details such as the title of the research, its aims/objectives, the context of the study, study methods, findings and conclusions, and relevance of the study to the present thesis.

Chapter 3: Research Methodology—In this chapter, various topics have been discussed such as research philosophy, data collection methods, research approach, type of research, and ethical considerations.

Chapter 4: Case Studies—This chapter reviews case studies on various ethical issues that are common for medical practitioners. The cases cover areas that include the following:

- Autonomy of the patients (respecting the decision-making ability of the patient)
- Discriminatory approach of the doctor
- Surrogacy issues
- Violation of the autonomy of the patient
- Ethical dilemma

The ethical issues in the case studies and their best solutions will be outlined. The method of case study analysis will be identifying the important facts and key issues, analyzing possible actions, and recommending the best and most suitable action.

Chapter 5: Survey Analysis—For the present research, we obtained primary data from a small survey. The survey was conducted with patients/their relatives regarding the virtues of the doctors and their approach toward their doctors.

Chapter 6: Discussion—In this chapter, a thorough discussion of the case studies, previous studies, and various theories will be conducted in the context of ethical issues in medical practices.

Chapter 7: Conclusion, Limitations, and Recommendations—The conclusion section will be a snippet of the entire research. The limitations of the research will be discussed, and various recommendations will be given for future studies.

CHAPTER 2

Literature Review

2.1. The Concept of Ethics and Bioethics

The word *ethics* originated from the Greek word *ethikos* that refers to the person's character. The word was then transformed to Latin, then used by the French (*éthique*), and finally translated to English. Kidder (2003) defines the term *ethics* as the "standard definitions of *ethics* have typically included such phrases as 'the science of the ideal human character' or 'the science of moral duty.'" In a nutshell, it can be said that ethics is related to the goodness and virtues of the human being and his nature of not harming anyone in performing the duty toward the human being and society.

The dictionary meaning of the term *bioethics* is "the study of ethical problems arising from biological research and its application in such fields as organ transplantation, genetic engineering, or artificial insemination" (Collins Dictionary). *Bioethics* is defined by Churchill (1999) as "the branch of ethics that investigates problems arising from medical and biological innovation." Bioethics is the combination of two terms: *bio* and *ethics*. Bioethics, therefore, is associated with ethical implications and applications of health science (*What Is Bioethics?* n.d.). Bioethics or clinical ethics work to identify, analyze, and resolve the conflict that arises when the service providers (physicians or doctors), patients, families, surrogates, and other stakeholders disagree on ethical issues or there is an ambiguity and uncertainty about the ethical practices (*What Is Bioethics?* n.d.).

2.2. History of Bioethics

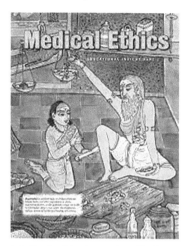

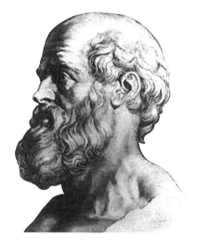

Medical ethics in ancient India
Source: Hinduism 2013

Hippocrates: Father of modern
medical oath
Source: Prioresch 1997

The history of bioethics traces back to the ancient civilizations such as Egypt, Mesopotamia, Greece, Babylon, and India. However, the researcher will focus on the modern history of bioethics, which starts pre-World War II. Nazi physicians and scientists of 1930s and 1940s were engaged in extensive human experimentation and resultant homicides during this period. In 1942, more than 38,000 physicians joined the Nazi Party in Germany and carried out unethical medical practices like the Sterilization Law (Jochen and Winau 1996). After the World War trials were conducted in Nuremberg, Germany, many of the physicians carried out inhumane and unethical experiments in concentration camps, which resulted in a stigma to humanity. The Nuremberg Code was passed in 1947. It included ethical principles such as informed consent and beneficence and was based on the Hippocratic oath. German physicians who engaged in unethical medical practices were tried. In 1948, the Universal Declaration of Men's Rights was published in which equality, freedom, right to life, and personal safety of the people were included.

Though the word *bioethics* was first coined in 1920s by Fritz Jahr (Sass 2007), the concept was scientifically put forward by American biochemist Van Rensselaer Potter in the book *Bioethics: A Bridge to the Future* published in 1971 (Whitehouse 2003). Just like the Nazis' unethical medical practice, one such unethical medical experiment was disclosed in 1972 in which the African Americans in Tuskegee, Alabama, were forced to participate in a study of the natural course of syphilis. These participants were completely unaware of their diagnosis of syphilis. In 1974, the National Research Act was passed under which the ethical principles and code of conducts were integrated. A commission was founded to conduct research on the status of bioethics. This commission called a meeting in 1976 to create a report on the fundamental guidelines. The resulting *Belmont Report* outlines three ethical principles: respect for the individual, beneficence, and justice. It was Beauchamp and Childress who proposed a fourth ethical principle by adding *nonmaleficence*. They replaced the term *individual respect* with *autonomy* (Mandal, Ponnambath, and Parija 2017). In the last few decades, bioethics organizations have developed and have produced guidelines for bioethics. Among these organizations are the World Health Organization (WHO) and its collaborating centers (CC), United Nations Educational, Scientific, and Cultural Organization (UNESCO), Council for International Organizations of Medical Sciences (CIOMS), Council of Europe, and Nuffield Council on Bioethics (Mandal, Ponnambath, and Parija, 2017). Today's ethics committees refer to these guidelines when approving various ethics-related cases.

The history of unethical practices from 1930 to 2003, and the response to such cases, has been presented by Kim (2012) in his research. In the following graphical representation, he focused on different medical scandals that took place in history and the response given to them (see fig. 2).

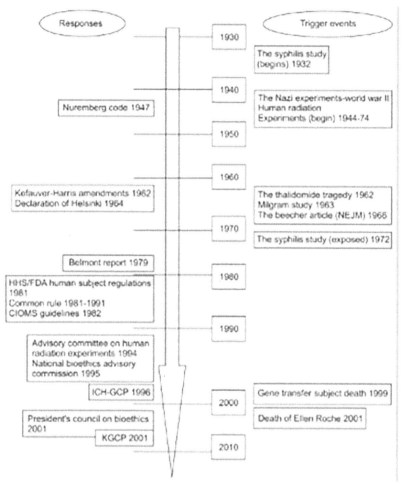

Fig. 2. Chronicles of scandals and responses to them. *Source*: Kim 2012

2.3. Ethical Decision-Making

Appropriate decision-making by physicians is very important for minimizing the cost and increasing the quality of the medical treatment. However, many times, making a decision is challenging for the doctors because it can involve several factors, outcomes, and complex relationships.

According to Beauchamp and Childress (2013), medical decision-making is based on the ethical principlism in which the guidelines are provided to make justified and correct decisions and to assess the morality of the actions. Each principle is prima facie, and each of them should be considered carefully (Rich 2019). As mentioned in the first chapter, there are four tools of medical ethics. These tools are used in the decision-making process as well. That is why it is crucial to find literature on these tools and their significance in the context of the decision-making process.

The first ethical principle of medical practitioners is patient autonomy. Autonomy is a core value of medical ethics (Varelius 2006). However, there is a debate regarding making decisions based on the patient's autonomy. According to some scholars, patients should not be allowed to make decisions if it is a question of their well-being and if their decision does not serve the purpose of their well-being (Buchanan and Brock 1990). The other opposite opinion is that in every circumstance, the patient should be given permission to make decisions regarding their health and treatment when the decision does not cause harm to anyone (Dworkin 1988).

Beauchamp and Childress (2001) opine that the doctors should certainly adhere to the ethical principle of autonomy if the patient is physically and mentally able to make a decision that is good for his/her health. But the authors also point out that allowing patients to decide and have freedom is not rationally or ethically acceptable if the patient is not in a position of making such decisions. The authors explain their reasoning by referring to the prisoners and mentally handicapped individuals, who should not be given autonomy. This means that autonomy should be given only if the patients meet certain parameters. While analyzing Beauchamp and Childress's idea of autonomy, Varelius (2006) elicits that if the person's choice is based on manipulation and coercion or if the autonomous decisions are based on false and inconsistent beliefs, he/she should not be given the autonomy to the make decision. In determining the patient's autonomy, it is legally and ethically obligatory for the medical practitioners to gain official consent from the patients prior to any risky treatments, but it is not unethical if the doctors do not inform the patients about the treatment if it is not risky (Dempski 2009). The doctor's decision-making regarding treatment is ethical if it is not harmful to patients' health and life.

If any decisions made by the doctors fail, it is the ethical responsibility of the doctor to inform the patients about the incorrect decision. Some medical professionals tend to make the decision to not disclose their error if it is not harmful to the patients. However, ethicists refute this decision, and so it is the ethical obligation of the doctors to disclose such errors. Thus, while making decisions regarding patient's health and treatment, the doctors need to be honest and transparent (Jonsen, Siegler, and Winslade 2010).

Beneficence and nonmaleficence are two other factors in bioethics and the ethical decision-making process. In this context, the research conducted by Swindell, McGuire, and Halpern (2010) is apt and relevant. The authors state that though the decision-making regarding treatment is dependent upon patients considering their autonomy, the doctors can use beneficent persuasion strategies to improve the patients' decision. According to the authors, it is the ethical responsibility of the doctors to help the patients make correct decisions. The physicians can use various techniques, which are as follows:

> Vivid depiction—Here, when the doctors want to change the decision of continued smoking by the patient, they can show him a video of patients with advanced lung cancer caused by the decision to smoke.
> Defaults—Evidence-based screening and making patients believe that the treatment is the only and default option.
> Regret—The doctors can help to change the incorrect decision of the patient by encouraging them to think about their regrets.
> Framing—Counseling the patients about their decision and the causal impacts on their health.
> Refocusing—Encouraging the patients to focus on their capacity to adapt themselves to the new life after their recovery from the severe injuries (Swindell, McGuire, and Halpern 2010).

While making an ethical decision, the physician is required to take into consideration whether or not his/her decision is causing any harm to the patient. It is the maxim, according to Beauchamp and Childress (2013), that "one ought not to inflict evil or harm." The principles of beneficence and nonmaleficence guide the medical practitioners in decision-making that would be for the betterment and well-being of the patient. Ethical decision-making in the health-care sector lies in making the decision that would be in the best interest of the patients. In ethical decision-making, the patient is and should be at the center of the decision-making process (Singh and Ivory 2015). Every ethical decision made by the medical professional needs to be considered with the utmost care. Being negligent and causing harm due to the decisions of the doctors can lead to an unethical practice (Rich 2019).

The decisions made by medical practitioners should be based on justice. When making fair decisions, the doctors have to take into consideration that every patient should have an equal right to receive appropriate treatment. The doctor's decision-making and subsequent treatment should not be contrary to the right of any patient. The doctor needs to include the principle of equality among the major criteria in the decision-making process in which there should not be any prejudice (Rich 2019).

Braveman et al. (2011) focus on some of the essentials of decision-making based on justice and equality. According to them, while making any health-related decisions, the doctors should treat every patient equally, think every person eligible to achieve his/her health status without any discrimination or marginalization, respect and follow human rights, make decisions that will not cause differences in socially deprived groups, make decision of distributing resources equally to every patient, and help to eradicate health disparities.

2.4. Ethical Challenges and Dilemmas

Ethical dilemma can arise when a situation occurs in which the decision-maker has to choose between two or more alternatives. It can prove to be an unpleasant situation when the choices are not simple because they cover a large number of principles (Figar and Dordevic 2016). Alkabba et al. (2012) shed light on the key ethical challenges that are faced by the health-care providers in Saudi Arabia. Their study revealed the top ten ethical challenges faced by the medical practitioners of that country. These challenges are patients' rights, equality of resources, patient confidentiality, patient safety, conflict of interest, ethics of privatization, informed consent, dealing with the opposite sex, beginning and end of life, and health-care team ethics. The top challenges faced by the doctors are the patients' right especially while giving them access to good treatment, receiving consent from the patients for any medical interventions, and confidentiality of his/her medical health. The second highest challenge is ensuring equality in accessing resources. According to the authors, it is the main problem in Saudi Arabia because all of the health-care facilities are concentrated in the large cities. The other eight challenges are also elucidated by the authors in this study.

The first pillar of bioethics is the autonomy of the patient. Ethical challenges are frequently associated with this pillar. Vaz and Srinivasan (2014) argue that a situation occurs when it is not possible for the doctor to give full autonomy to the patient for determining their treatment. The authors point out a situation in which sometimes the patients are suffering from acute psychological and mental disorders. Among them is schizophrenia in which the patient loses his decision-making ability. The same is in the case of dementia. In such situation, a conflicting and challenging situation often occurs. Mishra et al. (2014) conducted a study in which they observed bioethical challenges due to cultural differences. They found that the perception of individual autonomy is different in Western and Eastern cultures. Western culture is individualistic, whereas the Eastern cultures are collective (i.e., the decisions are made not just by the patients, but their families are also involved). Family participation is a major obstacle/challenge in ethical practices due to the cultural differences (Mishra et al. 2014).

Zubovic (2018) states that there are ethical dilemmas and challenges everywhere, in every primary health-care practice, and they are faced by both the nurses and the physicians. According to the author, ethical motivation and sensitivity play a key role in facing and over-coming the ethical challenges. The author also suggests that there be an integration of ethics in medical and nursing education. Zubovic explains the ethical challenges and dilemmas of the physicians and nurses in the form of decision-making about life, patient autonomy, justice, the conflict between the patients and physicians, professional-ism, truth telling, and religious and cultural reasons (Zubovic 2019).

In a study conducted by DuVal et al. (2004), it was observed that about 90% of the medical practitioners and doctors face ethi-cal dilemmas; however, the authors also confirm that the physicians overcome the ethical challenges because they have a wide range of skills, and they have resources and machineries available to them to deal with ethical challenges. The authors also strongly recommended that the health-care organizations should be persistent in integrat-ing deep ethical education in medical curricula. It was also the find-ings of authors that the ethical dilemmas faced by the physicians are based on their subspecialty, but end-to-end care is the most common ethical challenge among the doctors. Moreover, end-to-end care-re-lated challenges are faced more often by the critical care/pulmonary specialists than the oncologists. The primary health providers or the internists face challenges when their patients lack medical insurance and they receive limited reimbursement for the medical services they provide. Some of the physicians also encounter ethical challenges because they do not have access to any ethics consultation services (DuVal et al. 2004). About 19% of the physicians in the study stated that the ethical consultation services are not available to them.

2.5. The Qualities and Virtues of Physicians

The physician is the person who should act as a public servant. He/she should engage in a shared decision-making and healing relation-ship with their patients. It is very important for the physician to be active and empathetic in his listening and emotional ability. Only then will he/she be able to win the trust of his/her patients. Medicine is a moral practice according to Pellegrino, who identifies the virtues of the physicians as fidelity, trust, benevolence, intellectual honesty, courage, compassion, trustfulness, and practical wisdom. Pellegrino asserts that these virtues can be taught and inculcated. According to Shelton (1999), the physician is called "a good doctor" when he exercises respectful interactions with the patient and when he is an empathetic listener and appreciates patient's narrative. A virtuous doctor always acknowledges individualism.

The virtuous doctor as stated by Bain (2018) is always building a trusting relationship between himself and the patients, understands the feelings of the patients, and decides "the goods of the patient." According to Masel et al. (2016), the virtuous doctor or physician is an attentive listener. Moreover, he/she should be honest, experienced, gentle, and humane. The patient discloses many secrets to the physician. Hence, the physician should be a person with whom the patient can be comfortable in sharing the secrets that are essential in the healing process.

Considering the importance of virtues in a doctor's professional life, the British Medical Association (BMA) defines a doctor as a person with a fine combination of skills and virtues: "a set of values, behaviours and relationships that underpins the trust that the public has in doctors" (British Medical Association 2012). According to Cayton (2005), nowadays, patients are more concerned about the treatment they receive from their doctors. The patients expect that their doctors will treat them with respect, courtesy, and kindness. They should have good communication skills and the understanding of different options.

It was observed that the most common cause of the complaints of patients against the doctors is the lack of respect for their patients. It is the expectation of the patients that their doctors should be open and frank (GMC 2012). Respondents in the study believed that the doctors should be supportive, understanding, compassionate, and approachable (GMC 2012). According to the views of the final-year medical students, some core virtues need to be acquired by the doctors. These core values have been further segregated into subqualities (see fig. 2).

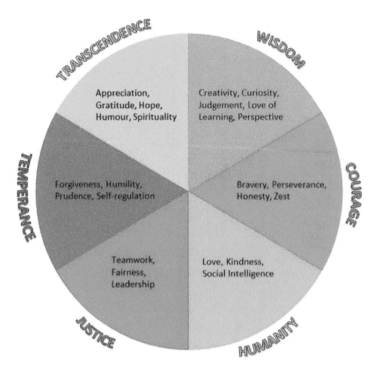

Fig. 3. Six core virtues. *Source*: Jones, n.d.

In the survey, the respondents perceived the attributes in the segment of courage (honesty) and justice (teamwork and leadership) to be most important, followed by humanity (kindness) and wisdom (judgment).

2.6. Doctor-Patient Relationship

In the health-care/medical profession, trust and communication are the fundamental factors for better treatment for the patients (Chandra 2018). This trust is either institutional or interpersonal. The interpersonal trust between the patient and the doctor can be developed through face-to-face communication and interaction. The access of appropriate and thorough information of the patients is required to be obtained by the physician. Along with trust and communication, a patient-centered approach is also a key contributor in improving the doctor-patient relationship. The better quality of services and mutual trust help to build a good concordance between the patient and the doctor. Trust and communication have been associated with patient satisfaction and health-care quality (Chandra 2017).

Shrivastava et al. (2014) state that the doctor-patient relationship is complex. This relationship is referred to by the authors as a contract in which the patient is expected to follow the rules and guidelines proposed by the doctor. A poor relationship has adverse impact on both the doctor and the patient and ultimately hampers the quality of health care. If this relationship is not healthy, the doctor and patient would not be able to treat the illness. When the relationship is poor, the patient does not have trust in the doctor, and they tend to change doctors repetitively and remain anxious (Shrivastava et al. 2014). They also observed that for the chronic lifestyle-related disorders, the patients usually try to keep a long-term relationship with the doctor. Because of this relationship, the doctors are fully aware of the history of their patients (Shrivastava 2014).

Stavropoulou (2012) calls the doctor-patient relationship a cornerstone of medical practice. It is a complex relationship where the patient and the doctor stand on two different sides. In this relationship, the doctor's treatment, prescriptions, and decisions determine the outcome of the patient's health. The patient in this relationship is empowered with making decisions related to their own health.

Charles (1999) studied the doctor-patient relationship in the context of three key models: paternalism, shared, and informed decision-making. In the paternalism model, the doctors diagnose the disease of the patient and decide the correct and most effective treatment for the patient. In this model, the doctor is the decision-maker, and the patient has a very passive role in decision-making process. In the shared decision-making model of the doctor-patient relationship, the doctor and the patient come together collectively to make decisions regarding the health of the patient and the appropriate treatment. Prior to the treatment, the patient and the doctor are in agreement with the treatment protocol, and there is a harmony in their relationship due to their collective decision-making. In the informed decision-making model, the doctors share critical information with the patient related to the health and the disease of the patient, and then the final treatment decision is based on the common agreement between the doctor and the patient (Stavropoulou 2012).

Chaix-Couturier et al. (2000) explain the doctor-patient relationship in terms of financial incentives. According to the research, there is a positive correlation between these two variables. If the incentive given to the doctors is less, they are likely to provide the minimum resources. However, this behavior of the doctors may affect their relationship with the patients. According to the authors, incentive is the motivating and determining factor for the healthy relationship between the physician and the patient.

There are some other factors that have an impact on a patient's perceptions of the doctor and consequently the doctor-patient relationship. In this context, Farber et al. (2003) conducted interviews with the parents of children suffering from asthma. They observed that the misunderstanding of medication can hamper a healthy relationship between the doctor and the patient. If the doctor is a specialist in the area, this misunderstanding is likely to decrease and the relationship improves.

2.7. The Ethics of Drug Use

Regarding the use/abuse of drugs, there are several social and ethical issues. Prescribing drugs is the responsibility of the medical practitioner. The quality and quantity of the drug are crucial. In his book, *A Layperson's Guide to Medicine*, Chowdhury (2000) has discussed some of the ethics that apply to physicians while prescribing drugs to the patients. According to the author, the drugs should be prescribed by the doctor rationally; and the focus should always be on rational therapy. It is ethical to prescribe essential generic drugs, which are a single-ingredient formulation with the accepted combination of drugs like co-trimoxazole, ORS, etc. (Chowdhury 2000). The author further suggests that when there are two or more options of drugs available, it is ethical for the medical practitioners to recommend the most cost-effective and safest alternative among them. In case of uncertainty about the dosage and side effects, the ethical practice is to refer to standard textbooks and/or journals. Apart from these, other responsibilities of the physicians according to Chowdhury are

- ➤ keeping themselves updated with the new knowledge by reading scientific journals and promoting clinical experiences,
- ➤ giving clear information to the patients about the drugs,
- ➤ explaining to the patients the necessity of taking drugs,
- ➤ not being involved in unethical practices of taking bribes and gifts from the drug companies or other benefits offered by such companies,
- ➤ avoiding cut practice and polytherapy, and
- ➤ trying to make the patient well in one visit (Chowdhury 2000).

2.8. Summary of the Literature Review

The literature review for this thesis was conducted on major topics related to medical ethics. The concept of ethics with its definition was discussed with the help of the previous studies. It is said that medical ethics are related to the goodness and the virtues of the physicians. It is important to have a strong conscience awakened in every medical practitioner. The history of bioethics/medical ethics was reviewed with the help of the previous articles and research papers. In the history, we reviewed the ethical background of medical science from the first half of the twentieth century. The unethical practices in the past were also reviewed. It was observed that the ethical codes became strict in a response to address and stop the unethical and inhumane practices that were prevalent in the twentieth century especially before, during, and after the World War II. We referred to the figure of chronological medical scandals that took place between 1930 and 2010. This graphical presentation was taken from the study of Kim (2012).

Previous studies related to the ethical decision-making process were also reviewed. The studies revealed that the four ethical principles are necessary to be considered while making ethical decisions.

These four principles are autonomy of the patient, beneficence, non-maleficence, and honesty. We also referred to the image of four pillars of medical ethics propounded by the previous studies. It was collectively found from the studies that ethical decision should always be patient-oriented, and the doctors should not make any such decisions that will harm the health and the life of the patient. Moreover, the doctors should be transparent and honest to their profession. They should respect human rights and equality.

However, it is difficult to follow the four principles of bioethics in every circumstance. In many cases, the doctors have to face dilemmas. So ethical dilemmas or challenges are also the issues that needed to be addressed. Considering this, the literature review focused on the previous studies related to ethical challenges that are faced by medical practitioners.

The attributes/qualities of the physicians were also discussed. Several studies have focused on different attributes the physicians should inculcate while doing medical practice. The major qualities are wisdom, courage, humanity, justice, temperance, and transcendence. The qualities of the doctors determine their relationship with their patients. With this in view, the literature review also focused on the doctor-patient relationship and its determinants.

This thesis will attempt to analyze different theories that are related to the medical ethics and their application in the medical profession. Along with the literature review and the theoretical framework, the case studies analysis will also explain whether the literature is complimentary. If there is any gap, it will be filled by analyzing different cases.

In the subsequent chapter, the research methodology used for this thesis will be analyzed thoroughly.

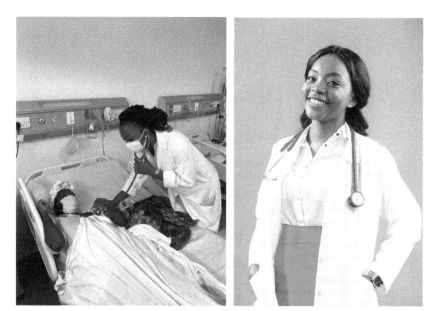

Dr. Esther Eghan, treating a patient in Greater Accra Regional Hospital, Ridge, Ghana.

CHAPTER 3

Research Methodology

The aims and the objectives of the research have been explained in chapter 1 of this thesis. The approach of the research must be complimentary to the aims and objectives. While investigating various approaches of research, the researcher has taken support from the study of Gibbons et al. (1994).

3.1. Research Approach

In the book *The New Production of Knowledge: The Dynamics of Science and Research in Contemporary Societies*, Gibbons et al. (1994) coined the terms *Mode 1* and *Mode 2*. Mode 1 is associated with scientific knowledge or fundamental research. It is related to the conceptualization of science as a separated discipline. Mode 2, on the other hand, is the sociology of science. While talking about the term *Mode 2*, Nowotny et al. (2003) stated that Mode 2 is "socially distributed, application-oriented, trans-disciplinary, and subject to multiple accountabilities." The present research comes under the category of Mode 2 in which our research is subject to multiple accountabilities of the doctors as well as being socially distributed and application-oriented research. It is application oriented in the sense that instead of teaching ethics in the classroom, it is important that the principles be inculcated.

3.2. Philosophical Paradigm

Considering these two modes, the approach of the present research is Mode 2 as it is based on problems that are transdisciplinary in the sense that it has its connection with other social sciences such as philosophy, medicine, sociology, economics, and cultural studies. Moreover, the research is also associated with many stakeholders (doctors, patients, nurses, community members financers, government, etc.).

There are two main paradigms: positivism and social constructivism. Table 1 defines the attributes of both of these paradigms.

Table 1

	Positivism	Social constructivism
The researcher	In positivist paradigm, the researcher monitors things independently.	The researcher immerses himself/herself what is going to be observed.
	Should be irrelevant	Key drivers of science
Explanations	Show interconnection	Based on the general understanding of the situation
Research progress	It is based on the formulated hypotheses and deductive method	Inductive method in which the ideas are explored from the accumulated data
Concepts	Need to be operationalized so that they can be measured	Integration of stakeholders' perspectives
Units of analysis	Simple in its analysis	Complex
Generalization	Statistical probabilities	Theoretical abstraction
Samples	Random sampling	Focus on the case study analysis

Adapted from Easterby-Smith et al. 2002

Apart from positivism and constructivism, the other fundamental paradigms are described by Zukauskas (2018) along with the ontology, epistemology, and research methods in the following table:

Table 2

Paradigm	Ontology	Epistemology	Research Methods
Interpretivism	Research and reality are inseparable.	Knowledge is associated with abstract descriptions of meanings formed by human experiences.	Case studies, interviews, phenomenology, ethnography, and ethnomethodology
Symbolic interpretivism	Research and reality intertwine.	Knowledge is created through social interactions and their resulting meanings.	Grounded theory
Pragmatism	The reality is ambiguous but based on the language, history, and culture respect.	Knowledge is derived from experience. The researcher restores subjectively assigned and "objective" meaning of other actions.	Interview, case study, and surveys

Source: Zukauskas et al. 2018

After studying the different paradigms of research, it can be concluded that the present research applies the social constructivist approach. In the research, the observer cannot be independent. Moreover, the researcher has not formulated hypotheses and attempted to test them. Sampling is also not conducted. The research is a theoretical abstraction. The topic *bioethics* is an abstract term, and the main focus of this research is on case study analysis. Interpretivism is also a philosophical paradigm of the present thesis as the knowledge in the thesis will be based on the abstract descriptions of the meaning gained through individual experiences (e.g., ethical dilemma, doctor-patient relationship, ethical decision-making, etc.). Moreover, like the interpretivism paradigm, the researcher has used the case studies for the thesis.

3.3. Problem Complexity

The problem complexity is associated with the ways to address the problems and searching for its probable solutions.

There are two dimensions to assess the level of the problem complexity. While discussing the problem complexity, Rasmussen (2011) has given two different parameters. These parameters are displayed in table 3 and table 4.

Table 3. Types of problems (Rasmussen 2011)

Problem	Characteristics
Type A problem	One or two parameters
	One field of knowledge
	Interviews/workshops
Type B problem	Some parameters
	One field of knowledge
	Intradisciplinary approach
Type C problem	A multitude of parameters
	Several fields of knowledge
	Interdisciplinary approach

Table 4. Domains of interests and value (Rasmussen 2011)

Domains of interest and values	Characteristics
Unitary	Stakeholders have similar interest and values.
Pluralist	Stakeholders have similar values but different interest.
Disparate	Stakeholders have different values and different interest

In table 3, three types of problems are mentioned. Research can be based on any of the three types. The present research is based on a type C problem. This is because the research consists of the knowledge of different domains from core fields such as medicine and philosophy. Moreover, it needs an interdisciplinary approach. This has already been discussed in the literature review. The topics such as history of bioethics, ethical dilemmas and challenges, and doctor-patient relationship and other such topics that come under the framework of ethics and philosophy have been covered in the research. Hence, type C is relevant in the context of the present thesis.

In table 4, the domains of interests have been included. In the context of this thesis, the second domain (pluralist) is appropriate. This is because the stakeholders have similar values, which are the ethics and welfare of the patients, yet different interests because the backgrounds of the stakeholders are different. In literature review, the Eastern and Western cultural interests have been mentioned.

Being a type C problem, it can be said that the research depicts interdisciplinary issues, has a conflict of interest, and has a high likelihood of disagreement on ethical issues (through ethical dilemmas), so it is sometimes difficult to find concrete solutions.

3.4. Research Methods

Research methods that are pertinent to this thesis include experiments, surveys, interviews, case studies, and archive analysis. Colotla

(2003) has explained the details of each method. The following table (table 5) shows the details of his work.

Table 5

Research methods	Types of questions	Requirement of control over behavior	Focus on contemporary events
Experiment	How, why	✓	✓
Survey	Who, what, where, how, how many, how much	X	✓ or X
Archival analysis	Who, what, where, how many, how much	X	X
History	How, why	X	✓
Case study	How, why	X	✓

Source: Colatla 2003

Based on the details given in the above table, the present research is a case study analysis with some aspects of history as well. The questions asked for the inquiry of the research start with either *how* or *why*. Examples are as follows:

➢ How did the concept of bioethics emerge?
➢ How should the doctor handle ethical dilemmas?
➢ Why is ethical study important?
➢ How can the doctor-patient relationship be cherished?

The focus of the research is on the contemporary issue that is ethics in the medical profession. Being the method of the present thesis, it is crucial to know what the case study method entails.

Case study is a common method used in social sciences. It is conventionally used for qualitative research; however, this methodology is also used for quantitative research and sometimes the combination of qualitative and quantitative methods. When defining the term *case study*, Sturman (1997) states that "case study is a general term for the exploration of an individual, group or phenomenon." Simons (2009) defines *case study* as "an in-depth exploration from multiple perspectives of the complexity and uniqueness of a particular project, policy, institution, program or system in a 'real life.'" This complexity comes from the change that is the resultant product. Case studies are based on a developmental factor in the sense that they evolve over a course of time.

Thomas (2011) classifies the case studies into different types: retrospective case studies, snapshot case studies, diachronic case studies, nested case studies, parallel case studies, and sequential case studies. According to Thomas' classification, it is vital to see which category the case study analysis of the present thesis falls. Retrospective case studies collect the data of past events and phenomena. In the analysis process under retrospective case studies, the researcher looks back at the past events and studies their historical context. For the analysis of the research questions formulated for this thesis, a historical review of the bioethics has been integrated by the researcher. Therefore, this thesis contains a few elements of retrospective studies.

In snapshot studies, the cases are analyzed and examined by considering one specific period of time. While conducting case study analysis in medical science, for example, in bioethics research, if the researcher intends to study ethical issues during World War II, it would be a snapshot study since the study focuses only on the period of WWII. The present thesis sheds light on bioethics in a modern context, but references from the past have also been considered. Having some elements of snapshot studies, this thesis is also classified as a partial snapshot case study.

A diachronic case study is a longitudinal study. The present thesis is also said to be a diachronic study. That is because the analysis of bioethics of modern time cannot be separated from the past events. To study modern medical ethics, it is essential to explore the past case studies as well. Hence, the researcher has followed the approach of a diachronic case study as well.

The present thesis cannot be called a nested study. This type of study includes a comparative analysis within one case, which are known as "nested elements." Considering the broader scope of the thesis, it cannot be studied under nested case study model. The thesis also does not follow the parallel case study or sequential case study approach.

3.5. Data Collection Process

In this section of the thesis, the researcher intends to focus on the process through which the data have been collected.

3.5.1. Determining Number of Cases

The number of cases in the research is usually determined by the context of the research. The case study analysis is conducted by taking a single case and multiple cases. The single and multiple cases can be either holistic or embedded. It is interpreted in the following table:

Table 6. Matrix of single and multiple holistic cases and single and multiple embedded cases

	Holistic	Embedded
Single	One case with one unit of analysis	Several cases each with one unit of understanding
Multiple	One case with several units of analysis	Several cases with several unit of analysis

Source: Adolphus, n.d.

In the present thesis, there are several subtopics that will be analyzed such as the background of bioethics, unethical practices in the past, ethical dilemmas/challenges, ethical decision-making in the medical profession, and the doctor-patient relationship. As a result, it is not possible to analyze all these different issues in just one case study. Hence, the approach for the present thesis will be a multiple embedded case study method in which several cases with several units will be analyzed. The major advantage of a multiple embedded case study is that the researcher can obtain evidence from multiple sources.

3.5.2. Challenges in Conducting Case Study Analysis

- ➢ Practical issues
  - o Confidentiality issues: The researcher attempted to contact the hospitals for finding case studies in bioethics, ethical practices, and ethical issues. However, most of the hospitals refused to give any case under the issue of confidentiality.
  - o Width, depth, and length of the study

- ➢ Validity
  - o Comprehension of the cultural, social, and economic factors involved in the case
  - o Maintaining objectivity as an observer or researcher
  - o Determining whether some of the components are practical in a modern context

The practical issues involved in the case study may result in delay of the entire research process. In the case of this thesis, it took several days to access the real-life cases from the hospitals. Sometimes, the case doctors were not available, and it was difficult to get an appointment with them due to their busy schedule. It also took several days to convince the medical authorities that the cases would be kept confidential and that the names of the doctors, patients, and hospitals would not be disclosed. The researcher had to spend a considerable amount of time in completing the process of obtaining consent from the stakeholders.

3.5.3. Selection of the Cases

Some cases were explored on the Internet. So it took substantial time to select the cases. The researcher contacted three local hospitals and chose three real-life cases. The remaining cases were obtained from the Internet. The cases were chosen based on the subtopics of the thesis (see table 7).

Table 7

Case	Topic	Details
Case 1	Doctor's discriminatory treatment to the patient	The doctor denies treatment to the patient after knowing that she was a homosexual person.
Case 2	An ideal case where the doctors followed all ethical rules	The case study of an elderly woman suffering from several fatal and complex health issues
Case 3	Violation of autonomy of patient but demonstration of beneficence	The doctors forcefully performed surgery on a woman when she had not given them consent to do so.
Case 4	Case of surrogacy	The couple hired a surrogate woman for implanting their egg and sperm. After the delivery, the surrogate woman refused to relinquish the baby to them, saying that she had an emotional involvement in the baby.
Case 5	Comparative analysis between two doctors. One was an example of a virtuous doctor, and the other was an unworthy doctor having some serious ethical issues.	Meghan was taking treatment from a doctor for her vertigo and imbalance problem due to which she had partially lost her hearing capacity. She shifted to another doctor due to some major issues with the first doctor.

3.6. Parameters of Selecting Cases for the Thesis

Prior to the selection of the case studies, the subtopics analyzed in the thesis were reviewed once again. The above cases were selected on the basis of the following parameters.

Unique and atypical example: The case studies chosen addressed at least one of the subtopics or issues covered in the subtopics and objectives of the thesis. It was also determined whether the case was a unique example of the problem and if the case provided new insights to understand and analyze the medical problems in bioethics context. Through the cases, the researcher realized various unique ideas of resolving the ethical problems presented in the case.

3.6.1. The Ability of the Case to Provide a New Insight to Resolve Problem

It had to be determined whether the case was able to provide new insights that result in the successful resolution of the problem. A case can shed light on the religious, social, and cultural contexts. For example, in case 4, it was observed that the doctor refused to offer the patient treatment because she was lesbian. This does not involve just a medical issue in this circumstance, but it encompasses the cultural, social, and human rights issues as well. The case will be analyzed thoroughly in the next section. It is referenced in order to show how new insights and dimensions of the issues can come to the forefront. That is why such case studies were perceived to be appropriate for the analysis.

3.6.2. The Ability of the Case to Pursue Action-Leading Resolution

While choosing the cases, the researcher also considered if the results and findings were derived in such a way that could help to resolve the existing problem as well as issues that may arise in the future. For example, in one case, a patient was admitted to a private hospital after a severe accident on the road. He was in critical condition. The doctor tried to save his life, but unfortunately, the patient died. The relatives of the patient berated the doctor badly. After this case, the doctor decided that he would never take accident cases in his hospital. Here, it is not important whether the resolution made by the doctor was right or wrong. The main point is that the case helped to pursue action-related resolution to the doctor.

3.6.3. The Ability of the Case to Offer a New Direction for Future Research

While choosing the cases, the researcher confirmed that the cases chosen could motivate future researchers to conduct research from a different perspective. For example, if the solution made in the case was not rational and logical, the researcher may recommend future study to find a better and more rational solution. Thus, the cases chosen for the analysis can be used for exploratory investigations, focusing on a more in-depth examination of the research problem.

3.7. A Generic Short Patient Experiences Questionnaire (GS-PEQ)

Sjetne et al. (2011) conducted a study on the GS-PEQ. In this type of questionnaire, the patients' experience was perceived to be the key outcome for the medical profession and the services it offered. To investigate the qualities of a virtuous and ethical doctor, a small survey was conducted with the patients of three local hospitals. In formulating the questionnaire for this thesis, the researcher considered the patient's opinion about the service and treatment and the overall approach of the doctor.

The data collection process was conducted by distributing a printed questionnaire. An online survey was not a feasible option as the researcher had approached the hospitals directly. So the researcher felt it was more feasible to distribute the questionnaire and collect the results from the participants before they left. That is the reason why the researcher managed to obtain responses from fifty out of sixty participants (83.33%). Had it been an online survey, it would not have been possible to obtain this high percentage of responses in such a short time span.

Patients were chosen based on the belief that they were in good condition to complete the questionnaire designed for the survey. The researcher did not offer the questionnaire to patients who were in critical condition or unconscious or not suitable to complete the form due to other conditions. The researcher preferred to query the patients from the Outpatient Department. The relatives of the patients were also allowed to participate in the survey. All the participants were assured that their identity would not be disclosed.

The generic questions asked were as follows:

Objective	Questions	Question types
To know the strong interactive skill of the physician	How much are you satisfied with your doctor's way of talking to you and asking questions about your health?	Likert type
To measure the trustworthiness of the physician	Do you have trust in the knowledge and competence of your doctor?	Close ended or yes/no type
To measure the caring nature of the physician	How much do you agree with the statement that your doctor cares for you?	Likert type
To measure the listening skills of the physician	Does your doctor give you enough time to talk to him?	Close ended
To know the people's skill and fairness of the physician	Do you have trust in the other staff members working with your doctor?	Close ended
To know the transparency of the doctor	Does your doctor communicate about the medicines they are giving you regarding their effects and side effects?	Close ended
To test "patient first" or patient-centric approach of the physician	Is your doctor available for you anytime when you need medical help?	Close ended
To measure the skill of physician to make his/her patient comfortable and relaxed and his/her gratitude and positive approach	Do you feel comfortable and safe when you are treated by your doctor?	Close ended

To measure trustworthiness and kindness	How comfortable are you while talking to your doctor? Do you feel that your medical information will remain confidential with your physician?	Close ended/Likert type
To measure humanitarian approach	How do you agree to the statement that your doctor respects you as a human being?	Band score
To know the compassion level	How would you rate your doctor for his/her compassionate level?	Band score
To know self-regulation and decision-making ability of the doctor	How would you rate your doctor for his/her decision-making capacity?	Band score
To measure communication skills	How would you rate the doctor for his/her communication skills?	Band score
Self-regulation	How would you rate the doctor for his/her commitment to you as a patient	Band score

- ❖ Close-ended question—The answer is expected to be yes or no.
- ❖ Rating questions—Rating from 1 to 5 in which 1 = worst, 2 = bad, 3 = average, 4 = good, and 5 = excellent
- ❖ Likert scale—Rating scale from 1 to 5 in which 1 = strongly disagree, 2 = disagree, 3 = neutral, 4 = agree, and 5= strongly agree

*Some of the questions are modified in actual survey questionnaire.

For this small survey, the random probability sampling method was followed. It is a method in which anyone (patients or/and their relatives) could be chosen. The questionnaires were distributed to 125 participants, and the researcher obtained a response from 110 participants. The survey was conducted on the hospital premises with prior permission from the hospital authorities. Prior to the survey, the participants were informed of the objectives of the research and the significance of their feedback so that there would not be any confusion or misunderstanding about the intention of the researcher.

3.8. Ethical Consideration

Ethics is the key component in every sector. While conducting research, it is important to follow ethical and moral principles. Ethics in research provides the proper guidelines to the researcher regarding how to conduct the research in a decent, sensible, and responsible way. Research is a publicly accountable process. That is why it is obligatory to adhere to research ethics. For the current research, the researcher has strictly obeyed the following ethics:

3.8.1. Honesty

Honesty and transparency have been maintained throughout the entire research process. Prior to collecting the primary data, especially from the hospitals, the researcher demonstrated immense honesty. The concerned authorities were contacted, and the objectives of the research were clear to them. While contacting the patients and their relatives, the researcher had a very honest approach.

3.8.2. Objectivity

Being objective in the research means being unbiased regarding any events or subjects. The researcher is unbiased in the interpretation of the results in order to demonstrate facts and not the personal opinion of the researcher. The researcher has shown fairness and was open to analyze all angles and perspectives of the phenomena. An objective researcher is like a judge, and being aware of this fact, the researcher attempted to take into consideration every aspect of the research questions. As a result, this research is a value-free research in a sense that it is free from any specific moral, economic, religious, and cultural stand. This objectivity has enabled the research to be reliable and trustworthy.

3.8.3. Respect for Intellectual Property

While collecting the data from the primary and secondary sources, the researcher showed immense honesty. Secondary data was obtained by reviewing the previous studies (literature review). The researcher has acknowledged the study of the authors by adding their names in proper APA parenthetical citations as well as in the reference list. The researcher is well aware of the copyright and plagiarism issues and, therefore, demonstrated utmost care while using the studies of the previous scholars. Moreover, the information has not been manipulated, fabricated, or misinterpreted. The thoughts of the previous authors have been mentioned realistically.

3.8.4. Confidentiality

There is a fine line between transparency and confidentiality. There should be a transparency regarding the objectives and the purpose of the study while dealing with the people associated with the research process. However, confidentiality is also very important, especially when the human subjects are participating in the research process. The names of the respondents (participants in the survey), the hospitals, and the concerned staff of the hospital were kept confidential. Thus, the participants are kept anonymous. The data obtained from the hospitals, doctors, and patients were kept confidential and used for the purpose of the research paper only.

3.8.5. Responsible Publications and Material

As mentioned above, research is a responsible process, and hence, it must be credible. To maintain the credibility and authenticity of the research, the researcher has strictly used academic publications such as peer review journals, books, and the articles from authentic websites. No other websites are used unless the information was universally true. While incorporating the articles and publications, it was first confirmed that they were from a reliable publication. The researcher has mainly used government websites (.gov) or the websites of university or educational institutions (.edu). The published books, journals, government websites, and websites of international organizations, such as WHO, UNO, and UNESCO, were relied upon as credible sources.

3.8.6. Respect

In the survey process, the participants are treated with the utmost honor and respect. The researcher asked them questions which were relevant and useful for the research objectives. Questions based on religion, race, and sexuality or other personal questions were not included. There were no offensive or contradictory questions or statements involved in the survey questionnaire. Moreover, participation in the research was voluntary. The respondents were not forced to participate in the research. They had full freedom to refrain from the research process. Prior to the distribution of the questionnaire, the participants were politely informed of the objectives of the research.

In the subsequent chapters, the theories of bioethics/ethics and morality have been discussed in detail.

CHAPTER 4

Case Studies

4.1. Introduction

The concepts surrounding case studies have already been discussed in the previous chapter. The case study model in research allows the researchers to analyze a situation or a specific event, investigate the issues, and determine the probable strategies to resolve the problems and attain the desired outcomes. In the health-care industry, case studies work as an instructive example so that the physicians will be familiar with different scenarios that they may have to face in the future. As stated by Crowe et al. (2011), the case study model introduces the physicians to in-depth and multifaceted complex issues in their real professional life. The case study analysis provides a broader lesson to the physicians. Prior to the analysis of the case studies, the researcher would like to explain how the case study analysis has been conducted for the present thesis.

1. Step 1: Focus of the discussion was determined.
2. Step 2: Selection of relevant cases. The researcher gathered cases from two local hospitals and from the Internet. In selecting cases, the subtopics have been used as a road map. The subtopics include the historical background of bioethics, modern ethics in medical practices, ethical decision-making, and the ethical dilemmas of physicians.
3. Step 3: Details of the case. The case was presented accurately.

4. Step 4: Discussion of the case. Major ethical problems were identified and discussed by applying ethical theories and models.
5. Step 5: Major findings were derived from the case.
6. Step 6: Strategies were suggested to mitigate the identified problems.
7. Step 7: The case was concluded with a succinct conclusion.

However, during the analysis, these steps are not followed in any particular order. Moreover, we have not made any effort to sectionalize them into the seven steps.

4.2. Case 1

This is the case of a woman who we refer to as Melisa (name of the patient is changed). She was admitted in the Helena Fertility Clinic (name of the hospital is changed). She wanted to become pregnant and had been trying to conceive for the last 2 years. She completed two cycles of in vitro fertilization as well as embryo implantation. Unfortunately, neither of these treatments proves to be effective. Melisa continued to be confident and did not lose her hope. She had trust in Dr. Billy, who was providing her treatment including sperm donation and implantation. Melisa was comfortable and open with Dr. Billy and felt that she could share anything with him. One day, she shared with Dr. Billy that she was homosexual and living with her girlfriend, Kate. She shared that they had been living together for the last 5 years and planned to raise the baby by sharing parenting. This new baby was going to complete their family.

Some days later, Melisa received a letter from Dr. Billy stating that he would no longer provide her treatment and that she needed to find another doctor. When explaining the reason for his decision, he wrote, "My conscience and my religious beliefs do not allow me to treat a homosexual person and the family of same-sex couples. I apologize, but I will not be able to continue your treatment." Melisa was shocked, hurt, and insulted. She immediately called his office. When the receptionist answered the call, Melisa raised her voice in agitation. "I want to talk to Dr. Billy." She told the receptionist about the letter. "Dr. Billy suddenly told me to find another doctor. I have been his patient for the last 2 years. How can he ditch me like this? He knows my medical history, and my records are here with him. How can he stop treating me now? You are welcome to tell him that I am filing a legal complaint against him to the state licensing board. It is discriminatory treatment, and it is not legal."

4.2.1. Discussion

The above case can be discussed from several different perspectives, which are as follows:

1. Doctor-patient relationship
2. Ethical principles (beneficence, nonmaleficence, autonomy, and justice)
3. Ethical dilemma
4. Ethical and moral duties of the physician

In addition to these perspectives, the researcher also intends to analyze the case through ethical theories of consequentialism and deontology.

4.2.2. Doctor-Patient Relationship

In this case, the doctor-patient relationship was initially extremely healthy. It is important to see which elements of a healthy relationship are present in the case. As stated by Raina et al. (2014), the important factors for developing a sound relationship between the patient and the doctor are communication, respect, confidentiality, professional honesty, and trust. The author further states that effective communication is the major determinant in developing and sustaining the doctor-patient relationship. Patients are customers who receive medical services from their physicians. In the previous literature review, it was noted that doctors who educate their patients, talk to them, and tend to be humorous and less formal are much closer to their patients than those who do not. Considering the time span of the relationship between Melisa and Dr. Billy and her deep trust for him, it can be assumed that Dr. Billy had successfully created and maintained a sound relationship with Melisa as his patient. Had there not been a sound relationship between them, Melisa would not have shared her sexual orientation with him since that is an extremely personal aspect of her life. However, on this one, single aspect of their relationship, we cannot conclude that Dr. Billy knew how to make patients comfortable and feel able to be as open and honest as possible.

A physician should respect the patient regardless of the patient's attitudes and background. It is not desirable for a physician to pass judgments on the color, race, gender, sexuality, language, or social status of the patient (Raina et al. 2014). Dr. Billy's behavior, in this regard, cannot be called ethical. With full trust in Dr. Billy, Melisa disclosed one of the most confidential facts of her life, thinking that knowing the background of her sexual orientation would help the doctor make better medical decisions. But Dr. Billy did not respect her lifestyle and her background. He defamed her by withdrawing medical care from her on the ground that she was homosexual.

4.2.3. Ethical Principles

The case also needs to be discussed from the perspective of the ethical principles of the medical profession and bioethics. In previous chapters, the concept of bioethics was discussed. As previously stated, respect for autonomy, nonmaleficence, beneficence, and justice are the four principles of medical ethics.

The issue of autonomy, or freedom of the patient, is not found in this case. As far as nonmaleficence is concerned, it is the ethical responsibility of the doctor to do no harm to the patient. Doctors must consider aspects such as the risk factors due to his intervention or nonintervention. The doctor should also ensure that he has ample knowledge and skill to treat his patient efficiently. One more important aspect of nonmaleficence is that the doctor should make it clear that the patient is treated with dignity and respect. Dr. Billy undoubtedly had an immense knowledge and the skills required to treat Melisa. Initially, he demonstrated respect and treated Melisa with dignity. Melisa did not have any concerns regarding the treatment she was receiving. Once Dr. Billy was made aware of Melisa's homosexuality, he abruptly stopped the treatment and made it clear to Melisa that he could not treat her anymore. Stopping treatment abruptly is certainly wrong and could have caused harm to Melisa. Dr. Billy failed to follow the principle of nonmaleficence.

The last principle of medical ethics is the justice. According to this principle, doctors should be fair and just while treating their patients. Every patient is equal and should not be discriminated against on the basis of race, gender, age, nationality, sexual orientation, education, financial conditions, and other such factors. Unfortunately, Dr. Billy did not follow the last principle either. He stopped treatment because Melisa was not a heterosexual person. He clearly exhibited discrimination against homosexual individuals. His behavior was contrary to human rights laws.

The case does not indicate whether there is an ethical dilemma. It was not mentioned whether Dr. Billy was experiencing a dilemma before making the decision to stop the treatment for Melisa. Hence, the researcher cannot comment about the ethical dilemma of the doctor.

The ethical factors are described in the following table:

Dr. Billy's evaluation in terms of medical ethics	Y/N/DN
Competence, knowledge, and skills	Y
His relationship with Melisa before knowing her sexuality	Y
He showed beneficence (giving good treatment to Melisa)	Y
He showed maleficence	N
Justice	N
Human rights	N
Ethical decision-making	N

Y, yes; N, no; DN, don't know
Dr. Billy's decision to stop treating Melisa is not ethical on several ethical principles.

4.2.4. Theoretical Consideration

As discussed above, the case can be analyzed by applying two theories of ethics: consequentialism and deontology. The consequentialist views about ethical action depend upon the results of the action (good/bad). The consequentialist theory is divided into three subdivisions: ethical egoism, ethical altruism, and utilitarianism. In ethical egoism, if the action/decision taken by the physician is good and carries positive results to the patient, it is a correct action. In ethical altruism, if the action is good for everyone, it is correct. The utilitarian theory states that if the action is good for everyone, the decision is correct.

Dr. Billy seems to be unsure whether his decision to not treat Melisa is good or bad. Had he been confident with his decision, he would have boldly and openly told his decision to Melisa face-to-face. Instead, he preferred to send her a letter. When Melisa called, he did not pick up the phone and talk to her directly. His action of sending a written refusal was an act of uncertainty regarding his decision. He might have felt guilty for not completing his duty as a doctor. Hence, from the ethical egoism perspective, his decision was not correct since it did not give him any assurance about its rightness and wrongness.

The second aspect of consequential theory is ethical altruism. Here, the well-being of other person is taken into consideration. "Ethical altruism is the love that cares not for its own; it enjoys acting for the sake of another's good without making this at all conditional on its impact on the agent's own well-being" (Pugmire 1978). If the action/decision of Dr. Billy had positively affected the well-being of Melisa, it would have been an ethical action according to the ethical altruism. But Dr. Billy refused to continue the treatment and caused Melisa distress. The abrupt and uninformed end of treatment caused Melisa grief. It was offensive, and she was hurt by the discriminatory behavior of Dr. Billy. It is not expected that a person should sacrifice his/her happiness for the sake of another's happiness. It is also not desirable to cause someone trouble. In a nutshell, Dr. Billy's decision/action cannot be ethical according to the consequential theory because the consequences of his decision and actions were not positive.

Some physicians refuse to treat homosexuals because they perceive homosexuality as a mental disorder (Drescher 2002). Dr. Billy gave the reason of religious conscience as his defense. It is quite possible that he might be thinking that Melisa suffers from a mental disorder. Some doctors exclude same-sex couples from fertility treatment because of the perception that the welfare of the future children may be compromised in the family of same-sex couples (Pennings 2012). Being a physicist, Dr. Billy was succumbed by old and outdated religious doctrines that science have already proved wrong. On the religious front, his action/decision may be correct, but from the perspectives of humanity and medical ethics (such as justice, beneficence, nonmaleficence, and justice), his action was unethical. It is also important to discuss what the law states and whether Dr. Billy's action was legal. For a thorough discussion, we have to take into consideration the American laws regarding the duties and responsibilities of medical practitioners in the United States.

4.2.5. Legal Aspects

The rights of the physicians are well protected in the United States. They have the legal right to refuse to treat the patient if they find it objectionable on an ethical or moral front. In the ruling of the Supreme Court in *Roe v. Wade* in 1973, the Church Amendments were passed in which physicians were given the right to deny treating patients in abortion and assisted suicide. Physicians also have the right under the conscience clause to refuse medical services on the ground of religion and their conscience. Along with abortion and suicide, doctors can also refuse treatment in the cases of sterilization, contraception, and stem cell-related treatments. On legal grounds, Dr. Billy's actions were lawful.

There is, however, a question regarding this legal privilege of the doctors because it restricts the patient's access to medical care.

In the case of Melisa and Dr. Billy, the doctor could have found a way to uphold his religious beliefs and Melisa's well-being. If he did not intend to continue his treatment, he could have referred the case to another physician. If this had been done, the dispute could have been avoided, and Melisa's access to medical treatment would not have been hampered. Fortunately, Melisa's case was not life-threatening. If the homosexual individual had a serious health problem and if Dr. Billy had refused treatment, he/she may have lost his life. The real ethics issue lies in providing treatment to patient, not the religious doctrines, which are many times irrelevant and impractical.

4.2.6. Patient's Autonomy

In this case, the patient's autonomy was respected. In the beginning, Melisa was happy and satisfied with Dr. Billy as he was giving treatment to her according to her wish. She wants to have a child, and respecting her decision, he took efforts to arrange sperms for her. He never performed any surgery or any medical activities without her permission. This autonomy developed a trust in Melisa's mind about her doctor that he was going to deliver best treatment to her. Melisa's complaint against Dr. Billy was not because he threatened her autonomy and freedom regarding her health, but her discontent was toward his approach that changed after he came to know about her sexual orientation. Therefore, we can conclude that Dr. Billy was ethical in respecting his patient's autonomy and freedom.

4.2.7. Conclusion and Recommendations

Based on the above discussion, the action and decision of Dr. Billy may be correct on legal grounds; but ethically, there are many issues to dispute. He failed to follow the principles of medical ethics. The decision-making of Dr. Billy was not practical but rather irrational. Sexual orientation and parenting are personal matters of individuals. They should not influence patient treatment. Human life is more precious than anything else in this world, and humanity is more important thing than religion. Even though his conscience did not allow him to treat Melisa, he should have ensured that she could access sound medical service under another skilled physicians. If cases such as this arise in the future, the following are some recommendations for physicians:

1. It is strongly recommended that when there is a conflict between the law and ethics principles, a virtuous doctor should prefer ethics to law and religion.
2. Religious beliefs should not come into play while treating the patient.
3. If an ethical dilemma arises, the doctors should first think about the life and well-being of the patients. All other issues are subordinate.
4. If, for any reason, the physician is not in a position to treat the patient, he/she should consult with other physicians and secure the right of medical access for the patient.
5. The ethical dilemma can be resolved by openly communicating with the patients and others.

4.3. Case 2

Ms. Merlin, an 81-year-old woman, was admitted to one of the private hospitals in the town of Australia. She had a fragility hip fracture after falling on the slippery floor. Apart from her physical injury, Ms. Merlin has been suffering from dementia for the last several years. Therefore, she is not able to make decisions regarding her own health. The physical movement of Ms. Merlin is limited, and she uses a walker. She was accompanied to the hospital by her two daughters, who informed the doctor that the health of their mother has been deteriorating for the last few days. Her confusion has increased, and she will not even come out of her room.

When the team of physician conducted their intake review, they found that Ms. Merlin had a pleural effusion (excess fluid) in her lungs. A heart murmur was detected during the medical assessment. Her heart was in very poor condition due to valve malfunctions. Performing surgery would have placed Ms. Merlin in a life-threatening situation with a significant chance of death.

Due to her age and extreme health complications, surgery would be too high of a risk for the patient.

The team of the doctors and the nurses encountered a dilemma in decision-making as they all had differing opinions of how to proceed. They debated and brainstormed on the proper action(s) that would ensure the well-being of the patient, causing no harm to her physical and mental health. The family members were anxiously waiting outside while the doctors debated. The medical team informed the family members that Ms. Merlin would not live without having surgery, yet due to her health and other complications, there was a great risk if the surgery were performed. The family also had a dilemma regarding the proper treatment for the patient. They could not agree on whether to choose palliative care or take the risk of surgery. At the request of the patient's relatives, the doctors explained palliative care and how it can be beneficial for the patients like Ms. Merlin. After a long discussion, the relatives of Ms. Merlin decided to proceed with palliative care.

4.3.1. Discussion

The patient involved in this case is an 81-year-old woman with a fragility hip fracture. She also has other severe and complicated health problems. The patient's relatives were extremely anxious, and the doctors were in dispute about how to proceed due to the deteriorating condition of the patient.

The focus of the discussion regards the best treatment for the patient that is both patient-centric and improves the welfare of the patient. This case is straightforward with no conflicts or disputes like case 1. That is due to the responsible and ethical behavior of the medical team. It is the objective to determine how the doctors follow the principles of medical ethics in this case. For discussing the case, the following principles of clinical ethics are taken into consideration.

4.3.2. Autonomy of the Patient

In this case, the participation of the patient is not possible due to her physical and mental state. She is not in a condition to make any decisions regarding her treatment because she has severe dementia. The decision-makers in this case are the relatives of the patient. The doctors had already informed them of the fatal condition of the patient. The doctors gave full autonomy to the patient's relatives to choose one of the following options: allow the doctors to perform surgery or pursue a palliative care option. The doctors respected the decision made by the relatives on the behalf of the patient. By doing this, the doctors followed the first principle of medical ethics—autonomy of the patient.

4.3.3. Beneficence

The term *beneficence* has already been defined and discussed earlier in this paper. It is an action that is carried out for the benefit of the patient. The doctors did everything that was beneficial for the health and life of Ms. Merlin. They ensured that Ms. Merlin had been given access to every possible type of medical assistance. They conducted all necessary medical tests during Ms. Merlin's hospital stay.

4.3.4. Ethics of Truth Telling

Truth telling is one of the key ethical principles of medical professionals. According to Zolkefli (2018), telling the truth is essential for the physicians. Truthfulness has a direct association with the ability of patients to make decisions regarding their health and well-being. The patient always expects truthful information from the doctor. If the truth is hidden from the patient, he/she cannot make an informed decision and give official consent for further treatment. Lying is perceived to be a breach of the autonomy of the patient (Zolkefli 2018). According to Kant, a philosopher, every human has a moral and ethical duty to tell the truth. He further states that the truth must be disclosed even though it is harmful and harsh (Kant 1964).

According to Jones (2005), the honesty and transparency of the patient help to protect the patient from overtreatment. In the case of Ms. Merlin, the surgery could be an overtreatment because it could lead to patient harm and additional complications. The doctors avoided every conceivable ethical issue with transparency and honesty. After thoroughly examining Ms. Merlin, they clearly communicated all health complications to the relatives since Ms. Merlin was not in position to make any decisions. They openly outlined the potential risk of performing surgery on Ms. Merlin. This transparency helped her relatives make good decisions.

4.3.5. Beneficence and Nonmaleficence

Under these ethics principles, the physicians are expected to carry out the benefits of others especially their patients. It is mentioned in the case that the doctors advised Ms. Merlin's relatives regarding the option of palliative care. They provided thorough information about palliative care and why it would be the most beneficial option for the patient. In similar cases, doctors can further take the step of consulting the patient and/or their relatives. It is because there are some factors which even the core doctors are not familiar with. They obviously conducted the interdisciplinary consultation with Ms. Merlin's family, but they can also suggest that patients take advice from an external expert or body if they wish. The ethical action is to carry out a meeting between the family members and the stakeholders to discuss the value of Ms. Merlin having either a meaningful life or a meaningful death. It can be easy for the family members to make the right decision by consulting the stakeholder.

As far as legal aspects are concerned, in almost all countries, the legislation and laws expect that doctors respect the decision of the patient or other decision-makers. This reflects a patient-centered approach.

4.3.6. Doctor-Patient Relationship

One of the key ethical principles of the doctor is to maintain a good relationship with his patients and their family members. This relationship was clearly established by Ms. Merlin's doctors with their well-mannered and ethical behavior. They included the patients' relatives in the discussions regarding Ms. Merlin's health issues, communicated her condition, and consulted the relatives regarding the potential actions that could be taken in Ms. Merlin's case.

Along with beneficence, Ms. Merlin's doctors also made sure that she was not being harmed by any surgery or operation. The doctors were trying their best to find ways by which the patient would get the least amount of pain, suffering, and harm. The following table summarizes the ethical behavior of the doctors through their actions:

Action of the doctors	Ethical principles
The doctors asked the family members of the patient what option should they opt for. Surgery or palliative care?	Autonomy of the patient
The doctors considered two different options for treatment and were brainstorming the possible treatments.	Beneficence
The doctors suggested the option of palliative care to Ms. Merlin because the surgery may have proven harmful.	Nonmaleficence
The doctors did not hide anything from the family members of Ms. Merlin regarding her health conditions. They openly explained that she had severe health issues.	Honesty and truth telling
The doctors did not bring any discriminatory issue during the treatment of Ms. Merlin.	Nondiscriminatory approach
The doctors had an ethical dilemma regarding the appropriate treatment. However, they consulted openly between each other and then later with the relatives of Ms. Merlin.	Sound doctor-patient relationship

4.3.7. Conclusion

Unlike the first case of this section, in case 2, there are no ethical issues or conflicts at any point. An ethical dilemma was present, but that was resolved through consultation with the patient's relatives. The doctors involved in the case demonstrated the utmost responsibility toward their patient and their commitment toward their duty of striving for the quality life of the patient. They were ethical on all fronts of the ethical principles. They showed immense respect toward their patient, and there were no legal issues involved in this case.

4.4. Case 3

A woman named "Maya" was admitted to the hospital. Maya was an erotic dancer by profession. On admission, she was having severe stomach pain. The doctor recommended that she undergo a CT scan. Through the scan, the doctor found that Maya had an abdominal aortic aneurysm (AAA)—a blood-filled bulge—that weakens the artery, and even normal blood pressure can be responsible for a rupture. A rupture can result in massive internal bleeding and extreme pain. In such a critical situation, there was no other option but to perform the surgery and correct the aneurysm as quickly as possible. The doctors warned Maya that they had very little time to make a decision because she could lose her life. But Maya was not ready for this surgery. She thought that if she underwent surgery, there would be scar that would almost certainly end her profession as a dancer. She firmly refused the surgery. The physicians pressured her, but she still remained extremely stubborn. The doctors knew that it was a life-or-death situation. It was necessary to get her medical condition stabilized. Despite being a life-threatening condition, she was refusing the surgery. This reflects that she could have an altered mental state. The doctors felt that she had a diminished state of mind, and they made a decision to conduct the operation. They did receive official consent from her. She was anesthetized; the surgery was performed and was successful. When Maya realized that she had been operated on by the physicians without her consent, she sued both the doctors and the hospital.

4.4.1. Discussion

Several ethical issues are involved in case 3 and will be analyzed by considering different principles of ethics. The key ethical issues of the case are the patient-centric approach, the autonomy of the patient, beneficence and nonmaleficence, and truth telling. Let's start the discussion with the four principles of medical ethics.

4.4.2. Patient's Autonomy

In this case, the doctors violated the rule of the patient's autonomy or freedom. It is a common and sensible expectation of a patient to be their own person and to live their life freely without anyone's control over it. There are several cases throughout history where the patients' autonomy was denied and their bodies were used for medical experiments. Beauchamp and Childress stated that a patient is free to make any decision intentionally and with substantial understanding. It is an ethical practice when the doctors are realistic with the patients regarding their health situation and then consult them for appropriate intervention. The medical authors have followed a liberal individualistic concept of autonomy "in which patients are regarded as the decision-makers and they make decisions and act intentionally, with understanding, and without controlling influences, external and internal, that determine their actions" (Stiggelbout et al. 2004). However, the patient must be allowed for those intervention. In other words, patient autonomy is a fundamental principle of medical ethics. But at the same time, this principle can be challenging in some critical cases.

In the case of Maya, the doctors made the decision to perform surgery on Maya when she was not ready for the surgery. She had already stated her decision, but her decision was not respected by

69

her doctors. Maya's surgery was a forced surgery. So it is absolutely true when Maya claims that the doctors violated the principle of patient autonomy. However, it cannot be concluded that Maya's doctors were involved in an unethical practice because they knew that if the surgery was not performed, their patient could have lost her life. Hence, they took a paternalistic stand, which will be discussed later in this section.

4.4.3. Beneficence and Nonmaleficence

Taking into consideration the life-threatening situation, the doctors provided the proper treatment to Maya that would be beneficial for her health and her life. Saving her life was the ultimate objective for the doctors. There were not any selfish or materialist issues involved by performing her surgery. By taking the action of surgery, the doctors promoted her well-being and prevented her from any life-threatening risk. Beneficence and nonmaleficence are the terms in which the physician strives to heal the patient through appropriate medical activities, and no selfish gain is involved in such activities. The doctors treating Maya perceived that it is their duty to save Maya's life at any cost. Hence, regardless of her refusal, they performed the surgery. Though the doctors violated the principle of autonomy, they have followed the ethical principles of beneficence and nonmaleficence.

4.4.4. Truth Telling

Maya's doctor did not hide anything from her. The truth-telling act can be explained in the context of Kant's deontological theory according to which doctors should never hide the truth from the patient in any circumstance, regardless of the consequences of telling the truth. Maya's doctors did not hide anything about her serious health issue. They openly told her that if the surgery was not performed, she would die. However, they deceived Maya by the forced surgery. Performing the surgery without her consent means they not have been open and honest with her regarding their intention to move forward with the surgery. There were no bad intentions involved in this surgery. On the contrary, their deception was ultimately for her well-being. There are several complications involved with truth-telling act in Maya's case.

4.4.5. Paternalistic Approach

Instead of a patient-centric approach, the doctors adopted paternalistic approach while making decisions regarding Maya's health condition. Raina et al. (2014) discussed the paternalistic/paternal or priestly model in the context of medical ethics. In this model, the physician acts as a parent or guardian of the patient. By using their expertise and know-how, the doctors make decisions. The ultimate objective behind this approach is to restore the health and to ameliorate the pain of the patient (Raina et al. 2014). In the context of the paternalistic approach, the study of Drolet (2012) is also relevant and important. The author talks about selective paternalism, which is used by doctors especially when the chances of shared decision-making break down.

Respect for autonomy is imperative, but shared decision-making and patient autonomy are not practical solutions in every circumstance. Sometimes, the medical decisions that are made by patients or their families are dominated by emotions, and there is the chance of inducing distress and confusion in their minds.

Maya's doctors initially tried to resolve the issue through a shared decision-making process. Accordingly, they pleaded with her to have the operation. They informed her about the potential threat. But when they found that Maya was stubborn, they decided to use a paternalistic approach and assumed the role of her parents or guardian. They showed disrespect for her decision to avoiding surgery because allowing her decision to stand would have been costly for the patient. They acted in the patient's best interest. Hence, their decisions and actions were not completely unethical.

4.4.6. Ethical Dilemma

The ethical dilemma involved in this case is how to be 100% ethical and follow all four principles simultaneously when those principles conflict with each other. If Maya's doctors had respected her decision and allowed her to leave and, in this process, she had lost her life, the doctors would have been blamed for not following the principle of beneficence. Here, the two principles (patient autonomy and beneficence) conflict with each other. Following one principle becomes a violation of the other.

4.4.7. Doctor-Patient Relationship

A sound doctor-patient relationship is associated with the virtues of the doctors and their persistence in clinging to medical morals and ethics. In order to establish a good rapport with the patient, a skilled and virtuous physician always exhibits good communication and interaction with their patients. The relationship rests on four major elements: mutual knowledge, mutual trust, loyalty toward the patient, and regards/respect for the patient. It is a fiduciary relationship according to Chipidza et al. (2015) in which the physician agrees to respect his patient's autonomy, maintain confidentiality, explain treatment options, and obtain informed consent. As background to these factors, it is important to know how and why the mutual relationship between Maya and the doctors became problematic and ultimately culminated in Maya taking legal action against the doctors and the hospital. The doctors used their mutual knowledge and shared it with Maya, who had full trust in her doctor. Her admission to the hospital indicated that she initially trusted the doctors. The doctors were also loyal toward Maya. They didn't give any discriminatory treatment to Maya, nor did they hide her health condition. They explained clearly the potential threat and the need for an urgent surgery. However, they did commit an ethical error for not obtaining informed consent from the patient. This is the most important part of the case and is why the case defies medical ethics.

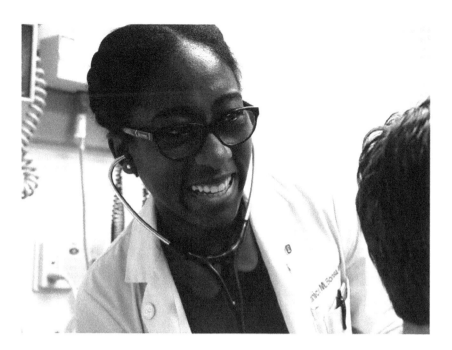

4.4.8. Legal Aspects

The supreme courts of almost all states in the United States as well as other countries have focused on patient consent as an ethical imperative. For example, the New York State Supreme Court held, "Every person of adult years and sound mind has the right to determine what shall be done with his own body and a surgeon who performs an operation without his patient's consent commits an assault for which he is liable in damages" (Schloendorff v. Society of New York Hospital 1914). However, under the emergency exception, immediate intervention can be applied without formal consent if not performing the surgery would lead to the death or serious physical damage to the patient. On legal front, the decision of Maya's doctors may be considered legal under the emergency exception term.

In the below checklist, Maya's doctors have been evaluated based on several ethical grounds.

Principle of bioethics	Whether followed by Maya's doctors Yes/no	Proof/incident
Autonomy of the patient to make decision	No	Without her official consent, they performed a major surgery.
Respect for the patient	No	They made a hasty perception that Maya had a compromised state of mind.
Beneficence	Yes	They operated on Maya to save her from the deadly condition that would have caused her death.
Nonmaleficence	Yes	They tried to make no harm to their patient at any circumstances.
Justice	Yes and no	They avoided causing harm to her health but not to her freedom.
Truth telling	Yes	The physicians warned her that if the surgery was not done urgently, she could lose her life.
Doctor-patient relationship	Troubled	It is because of the deceptive act of the doctors.

4.4.9. Suggested Ethical Recommendations

After a thorough review of the case, the researcher would like to suggest some recommendation to avoid any such situations in the future. Firstly, the doctors' opinion about Maya's state of mind was haste and without any proof. They did not have any medical record or evidences available with them that can prove that Maya's mental condition was not good. It is not mentioned in the case that Maya had any mental or psychological problem. She was refusing surgery because of her concern that the surgery would affect her professional life. It was not because she had any acute psychological imbalance. It was the big mistake committed by the physician in the case of Maya.

Instead of performing a forced surgery on Maya, the doctor should have convinced her that the surgical scar was not as big of an issue as she was thinking. Through counseling and consultation, the doctors could have removed any incorrect perceptions from her mind. The option of cosmetic surgery was available to hide the scar. Sacrificing her entire life for the sake of a scar was a very irrational thought. It was possible that she was refusing the treatment because of anxiety due to such a sudden and life-threatening health problem. So the option of consultation and counseling was available through the doctors. The question remains whether there was enough time for consultation and counseling because the surgery was extremely urgent. Giving the option of cosmetic surgery to hide the scar was a feasible alternative for the doctors to propose instead of performing surgery on such a war foot basis. The doctors should have adopted a paternalistic approach but in a more sober way by pampering and convincing Maya. Because of one decision (right or wrong), the doctors lost the trust of the patient. The reputation of the hospital was also affected, and the doctors would need to undergo a time-consuming legal process and will likely be served with a large monetary fine if they fail to convince the court that their intentions were appropriate.

4.5. Case 4

This case was narrated by a doctor in one of the local hospitals that the researcher visited for the purpose of research. In keeping the patient's anonymity, her real name has been changed.

Kate was diagnosed with uterine cancer and had to undergo a hysterectomy. Prior to her surgery, the doctor removed several eggs from her ovaries so that she could have the possibility of having a baby in the future. After the surgery, she was married and started a family with her husband. The couple decided to have a baby of their own. Since it was not possible for Kate to carry the child, the couple met with the doctor for a consultation regarding surrogacy. After procuring sufficient information from the doctor, the couple contacted a company that could provide them a surrogate mother. The husband's sperm and one of Kate's eggs were used for the fertilization. The sperm and the egg were implanted in the surrogate mother hired by the couple. The couple paid $20,000 to the surrogate and bore all expenses of her hospitalization, medication, and other medical tests. The couple spent a total amount of $35,000 during the pregnancy. They also paid $6,000 to the company that arranged for the surrogate. They were ensured that proper care was taken of the surrogate mother during her pregnancy. Kate and her husband were eagerly awaiting their baby. Everything was going smoothly. The surrogate mother gave birth to a healthy baby boy. Kate and her husband were very happy that finally they had their own baby. They had gone through much trouble for the baby. Their dreams had come true. But soon, they realized that their dream of having a baby was about to be taken from them. The surrogate announced that she could not give the baby to them because she had become extremely attached to the baby, and she referred to him as "her" baby. A legal battle ensued between the surrogate woman and the couple.

4.5.1. Discussion

Surrogacy is a widely discussed topic throughout the world. It is controversial as it consists of legal, ethical, and emotional factors. There is a couple who is not fortunate enough to have their own baby due to medical issues. Instead of adopting a child (who is not their biological child), some couples prefer the option of surrogacy. They are insistent on having their own biological child. The concept of surrogacy emerged from this desire. Surrogacy is a boon for both heterosexual and homosexual couples. From the above case, the readers come to know the concept of surrogacy, which is a provision/contract between a woman and a couple that wishes to have the child of their own. The woman hired as a surrogate mother carries the baby, which is not biologically hers. It is expected that once the child is born, the infant will be surrendered to the couple as per the contract.

This case is a commercial surrogacy case in which there was a clear contract between the surrogate and Kate and her husband. The contract must be written and signed by both parties.

The surrogacy contract and its legality vary within American states. Some of the states (such as Arizona, Colorado, Michigan, etc.) do not recognize surrogacy contract, while some states (such as Akansas, Florida, Ohio, etc.) do favor the surrogacy. In many states, there are no statutory provisions regarding surrogacy.

The laws regarding surrogacy are different in other parts of the world. Commercial surrogacy is legal in some US states, India, and Ukraine, while it is illegal in other US states, England, and Australia (Saxena 2012). In some European countries such as Norway, Germany, and Sweden, there is no legal recognition of the surrogacy agreement. In India, the surrogacy process is relatively easy and not very expensive.

The above case took place in a state where the laws are favorable for surrogacy. The couple found a proper surrogacy center, completed all procedures, paid the company, and hired the woman for surrogacy. So from a legal perspective, the situation is favorable to Kate and her husband.

Let's consider the case from the ethical dimension. Kate and her husband wanted a biological child. But due to medical reasons, they needed to engage a surrogate to carry the pregnancy. They provided their sperm and egg for the conception of the baby. There is no denying that the couple were the biological parents of the newborn baby. The surrogate mother had no biological relationship to the baby. Kate and her husband bore all expenses during the surrogate's pregnancy and had given her considerable compensation. They had put great effort into conceiving a baby and making legal and proper arrangements for its care. When there is a contract between two parties, there is no room for emotion. At the inception of the contract, the surrogate mother should have realized that the child was not going to belong to her after the birth. Being cognizant of this, she believed that she was ready for surrogacy and that regardless of her emotions, she must abide by the terms of the contract. Even though she became emotionally attached to the baby, Kate and her husband had an equal emotional attachment. One other important factor that cannot be overlooked is that she was a professional surrogate mother. It was her profession, and she was associated with the company for the same purpose. Hence, her claim of being emotionally attached to the child cannot withstand legal muster.

According to some scholars, surrogacy is like prostitution. When comparing these two professions, Prokopijevic (1990) states, "In both cases one's physical service is being offered, in both instances a deep personal or emotional relationship is not required for the transaction to be completed, in both cases material compensation is offered for the physical services provided." The opponents of surrogacy criticize it as a form of exploitation of female body, which is similar to prostitution (Warnock 1985). In surrogacy, the surrogate woman has to forget that she is pregnant and going to deliver a baby. She is just a "human incubator" for someone's child.

As defined by Warnock (1985), surrogacy cannot be argued as an exploitation of female body in this case. There was no compulsion on the surrogate mother to bear the child for the couple. Had she refused earlier, the couple would have found another surrogate. For the couple, it was a business transaction, and they were professional in their approach. They never went against humanity. They never forced her to carry their baby for them. The surrogate woman was free to make her own decision. After her consent, the couple use their sperm and egg to conceive a child. Furthermore, as stated by Prokopijevic (1990), an emotional relationship is not required for there to be a contract. While making a legal agreement, there is no place for emotion. Purely for the sake of pampering the emotions of the surrogate woman, it can be ethical and justifiable to give the child to her.

The couple was very honest and transparent with the surrogate woman. They took care of her. In the beginning while making a contract with the couple, the surrogate clearly knew that although the child would be growing in her womb, she was not the mother. Everything was clear. The couple paid the agreed-upon amount. On a biological front, the baby belonged to Kate and her husband.

Hence, the surrogate cannot claim the child. The potential loss for the couple is much higher than the loss of the surrogate.

However, the surrogacy procedure is a debatable practice relative to several issues such as money/payment for services (payment), gender (this profession is exclusively for women, and men can never enter in this profession), and exploitation. These three points need to be discussed in the context of the case. Surrogacy is a profession like any other profession in that it involves labor in both the sense of the body and the emotions of the individuals involved in surrogacy process. The ethical dilemma is this: If the business involves emotions, can it be called a profession? And if it is not a profession, should the intended couple pay the surrogate mother? There is money involved in surrogacy; hence, there should be a practical approach from both sides. Conversely, from the perspective of the surrogate, emotions should not be overlooked. Usually, women are quite attached and sometimes sensitive about their reproductive systems. So pregnancy is a special phenomenon in their life. Their commitment and attention to the pregnancy cannot be denied. Moreover, the surrogate has given birth to a living baby, not a doll. Another important aspect is whether the surrogate woman attains autonomy over her body when it is used for the purpose of surrogacy. In this case, autonomy was fully maintained. The surrogate woman was not forced or pressured during her pregnancy.

As mentioned previously, the laws of surrogacy differ from country to country. There tend to be two different views regarding the issue. In some countries, the surrogate is regarded as the legitimate mother of the baby, whereas in other countries, the biological mother is considered the legitimate mother. The laws of the state in which this case took place are favorable to surrogacy; hence, the chances the couple retaining their rights to the child are high. It is recommended, however, prior to using surrogacy, couples should first study the laws of the respective state or country thoroughly and then make their decision. The following factors should be taken into consideration prior to the decision:

1. Whether the law is favorable to surrogacy. If it is legal, the intended parents keep themselves safe.

2. Whether the contract/agreement of surrogacy is in alignment with the law.
3. Whether the surrogate is voluntarily ready for surrogacy.
4. It is also highly recommended that the intended couple consult an attorney about the potential risks involved in surrogacy.

4.5.2. Conclusion

After thorough discussion regarding the ethical issues in surrogacy, several points come to the forefront. The dispute and conflict in the case is who will be the legitimate mother of the child—Kate or the surrogate mother? On the grounds of transparency, honesty, autonomy, human rights, and finances, Kate and her husband followed all ethical practices. Moreover, they respected the surrogate woman, took care of her, and provided her the best treatment. The child that had been growing in the womb of the surrogate woman was their biological child. The surrogate was free to make her decision prior to the contract. The laws of the state in which this case happened was in favor of surrogacy. In this case, the basic bioethics were followed by both parties involved. The problem was with the surrogate's changing stance, which was shocking and disturbing for the couple. Even if this case were discussed front its emotional aspects, Kate is more vulnerable than the surrogate. This is because she had realized her dream of having a baby. Suddenly, her dreams were shattered by the deception of the surrogate, who previously agreed to this process and broke the contract in spite of being paid. On ethical grounds, the surrogate mother should relinquish the baby to Kate and her husband and adhere to the contract. State laws are in favor of the couple, and with the help of an attorney, they should be able to gain the legal custody of their child. In the future, other intended parents should take a lesson from this case and clearly outline all parameters before entering into such a contract, paying special attention to what to do if a conflict arises.

4.6. Case 5

Meghan was a well-educated woman working as a college professor. She had a problem with dizziness and vertigo. She visited an ear, nose, and throat (ENT) specialist because the dizziness was due to the imbalance in the fluid of her inner ear. During the first few visits, the physician, Dr. Phoebe, was fine although Meghan felt that she was arrogant and dominating. Meghan thought that it might be her nature and approach, so she did not pursue it further. After several visits, she came to know that Dr. Phoebe's thoughts were not on her symptoms during the visit. Dr. Phoebe talked on a phone for a long time with her family members, leaving Meghan sitting and waiting for half an hour. After her phone call was over, Dr. Phoebe continued to talk about her daughter and husband and their family function instead of discussing Meghan's health. One day, Meghan could not hear what Dr. Phoebe was saying due to the partial hearing loss, and she requested that Dr. Phoebe repeat what she said. Dr. Phoebe raised her voice and responded in a very rude way. Meghan was disturbed and offended. But she was a calm and sensible person and did not like to get into any kind of quarrel. Furthermore, Meghan had observed that Dr. Phoebe was emphasizing allopathic medicines with high dosages. She talked to Dr. Phoebe about that, but Dr. Phoebe told her that considering the severity of her imbalance problem, she needed a heavy dose. After taking the prescribed dosage, Meghan would feel better for a while. However, if she forgot to take the medicine, she felt dizzy again. Meghan wanted to be a normal person without taking any medicine.

Meghan decided to seek a second opinion. A friend told her about a local vertigo specialist named "Dr. Smith." Meghan made an appointment and visited his clinic. Unlike Dr. Phoebe, Dr. Smith was an extremely approachable, amiable, and loving person. Meghan briefed him on her condition. He was very empathetic and listened to Meghan attentively, so much so that Meghan felt like she had known him for a long time. He conducted some medical tests in his clinic such as audiometry, videonystagmography (VNG), rotation test, head impulse tests, etc. He eased her mind by saying that there was nothing seriously wrong, and the problem could be solved through proper exercises. Dr. Smith prescribed a small tablet with a low dose and told her to come back 3 days later. Meghan felt better due to this medicine. During her second visit, the doctor taught Meghan exercises for her eyes, neck, back, shoulders, etc. and insisted that Meghan do them on daily basis. After 8 to 10 days, Meghan felt totally free of the dizziness. Dr. Smith has become Meghan's doctor and friend. They have discussions on several topics in both the educational and medical fields. He also proposed to Meghan that they should write a research paper by combining medicine and education field. Meghan was very excited with the proposal.

She has not seen Dr. Phoebe or any other ENT specialist for the past 5 years. She has been seeing Dr. Smith once a month for routine checkups. She trusts him, and they have a very good relationship. One day while reading a review about Dr. Smith on the Internet, she found that the average rating of Dr. Smith's medical service was 4.9 out of 5. "It is expected," she said and smiled.

4.6.1. Discussion

The case analysis describes the quality of a virtuous doctor. It is a comparative analysis between two doctors. Prior to the analysis, it is vital to discuss the qualities of a good doctor. A good doctor needs to acquire core skills as well as other essential skills. Through core skills, it is mandatory for the doctor to have a thorough knowledge of his respective area. Apart from knowledge and expertise, the doctor should inculcate some virtues such as compassion, understanding, empathy, listening skills, honesty, commitment, and sound communication skills.

When Meghan visited Dr. Phoebe's clinic, the doctor did not seem to be approachable. As stated by Meghan, she was aggressive and arrogant. Merely prescribing medicine was not enough for the patient, but rather, Meghan needed psychological support and motivation from the doctor. Doctors should demonstrate a positive approach and keep the patient balanced. Many times, depression and anxiety can be the cause of vertigo issues. Dr. Phoebe should have understood that due to imbalance and dizziness, the patient lost confidence. In such a situation, Dr. Phoebe's arrogance caused even more depression for Meghan. Instead of building Meghan's confidence, Dr. Phoebe told her that her dizziness and balance issues were so severe that she needed a heavy dose of medication. By doing so, she created a fear of a disease process in Phoebe's mind.

Conversely, Meghan found Dr. Smith to be extremely approachable. He listened to her symptoms thoroughly, asked questions, and obtained more information from her. He demonstrated full commitment toward Meghan. He told her that she did not need to be afraid of having a disease since her problem was not serious. During healing process, the doctor-patient relationship is imperative. If this reciprocal relationship is maintained, the patient will gain confidence in the doctor and the treatment process. Dr. Smith demonstrated immense compassion and consideration, which made the patient feel as if the doctor was taking care of him/her on personal level.

4.6.2. Listening Skills

The major difference that Meghan observed between Dr. Phoebe and Dr. Smith was their listening skills. Dr. Phoebe did not seem to be interested in her patients and their problems. As mentioned by Meghan, Dr. Phoebe talked to her family members for a long time while the patient was waiting for her intervention. She was least concerned about the patient. Instead of discussing the patient's health, she discussed her own family and personal life. Due to such a disruptive interaction with the patient, the doctor could not develop an effective treatment plan for the patient due to her lack of attentiveness. Conversely, Dr. Smith made Meghan feel relaxed on the first visit. He was so attentive that Meghan could openly talk to him and discuss her symptoms and the history of her disease.

4.6.3. Commitment

Dr. Smith was committed to his patient as is seen particularly in his approach of focusing on nonpharmacological therapies and exercises rather than pharmacological intervention or medication. He spent substantial time training Meghan to do different exercises that could relieve her balance and vertigo problems. Dr. Phoebe could have taken this approach since she was one of the most reputable doctors in the town. Instead, her focus was on pharmacological intervention with a heavy dosage. Dr. Phoebe never suggested any kind of therapeutic exercises. This indicates that Dr. Smith was committed to his profession and to the well-being of his patient. Dr. Smith also demonstrated beneficence while treating Meghan. Taking the patient out of the vicious cycle of allopathic medicine is probably the greatest success of Dr. Smith. A virtuous doctor is always persistent about exercising for good health instead of just being treated with medication.

4.6.4. Nonmaleficence and Respect

Nonmaleficence means not doing any harm to the patient. Harm is not always a physical attribute, but rather, it can be mental or psychological as well. Making offensive comments about Meghan's hearing loss, raising her voice, and talking in a rude tone are hurtful to the patient. It caused a great deal of psychological and mental stress to a patient who was already panicky and anxious. Though Meghan did not have training in the medical field, she was well-educated, talented, and worked in a prestigious profession. Dr. Phoebe should have respected Meghan's knowledge and education. Meghan had every right to ask Dr. Phoebe whether it was necessary to take such a heavy dose of the medicine and to inform the doctor that she would prefer a nonmedicinal approach. Dr. Phoebe should have given her a more professional explanation of her reasoning for the need of medication. Dr. Phoebe did not take the patient's desires into consideration when issuing her opinion. In short, she was disrespectful of Meghan's wishes.

When talking to Dr. Smith, Meghan never felt any embarrassment. He respected her education and knowledge. He also took an interest in finding out more about her education and work specialization. In this way, Dr. Smith respected Meghan both as a person and as a scholar.

4.6.5. Comparative Analysis

A comparative analysis between Dr. Phoebe and Dr. Smith is presented in the following table:

Virtues/qualities of the doctor	Dr. Phoebe	Dr. Smith
Compassion/ kindness	Dr. Phoebe was rude, arrogant, and unapproachable.	Dr. Smith was compassionate and approachable.
Beneficence	Dr. Phoebe did not think that the prolonged heavy dose of medicine could have an adverse impact on Meghan's health.	Dr. Smith carefully conducted required tests and found the best option for intervention for Meghan based on her wants and needs.
Respect	Dr. Phoebe never considered that Meghan was also a leader in her profession and, therefore, should be respected for her education and knowledge. Most importantly, Meghan should be respected and treated like a human being. Dr. Phoebe insulted Meghan and had a negative attitude toward her.	Dr. Smith respected Meghan as a scholar and as a person. They discussed a variety of topics that he acknowledged Meghan's knowledge and talent.
Trust	Dr. Phoebe could not build or retain the trust of Meghan, causing Meghan to seek treatment elsewhere.	Dr. Smith was a skilled doctor, who could easily win the trust of his patient.

Commitment level	Extremely low (Dr. Phoebe was more interested in her family affairs than the patients' health)	Extremely high (Dr. Smith was giving the best treatment with his full commitment)
Doctor-patient relationship	Due to the negative attitude and treatment approach of Dr. Phoebe, she could not engage in a reciprocal relationship with her patient.	Due to the kindness and empathetic approach of Dr. Smith, he could develop a very sound relationship with Meghan and other patients.

4.6.6. Conclusion

Based on the discussion above, it can be concluded that the patient expects good care and a positive approach from the physician in addition to a comprehensive treatment protocol. Patients expect that the physician should be virtuous and trustworthy. A virtuous doctor should consider nonpharmacological as well as pharmacological treatments. Compassion, commitment, respect for the patient, listening skills, sound communication, and trustworthiness are all prerequisites of a virtuous doctor.

The virtuous doctor (Dr. Smith) proved that there is healing power not just in medicine but also in genuinely caring for the patient. Dr. Smith was the epitome of a virtuous doctor. On the contrary, Dr. Phoebe was an example of an unethical doctor. Dr. Phoebe demonstrated her purely commercial and indifferent approach in treating with Meghan, whereas Dr. Smith showed extreme compassion and dedication toward his patients.

CHAPTER 5

Survey Analysis

The researcher conducted a survey of patients to identify what ethical qualities and virtues they believed to be important in a successful physician. The survey was conducted with patients from several different departments within the hospital. The data obtained does not reflect the virtues of any one doctor in particular, but rather, it is generic data. The aim of collecting such nonspecific data is to gain insight of the most important aspects of medical ethics from the standpoint of the patient. As mentioned in the research methodology chapter, the questionnaires were completed by 110 participants.

5.1. Communication Skills of the Doctor

Question 1 sought to understand the importance of the interpersonal and communication skills of the physician. The participants were asked whether their doctors asked them questions about their health in an understandable way. A Likert scale was used to measure the results. The following table summarizes the responses of 110 participants:

Statement	Very satisfied	Satisfied	Neither satisfied nor dissatisfied	Dissatisfied	Very dissatisfied
How much are you satisfied with your doctor's way of talking to you and asking questions about your health?	76	13	10	1	1

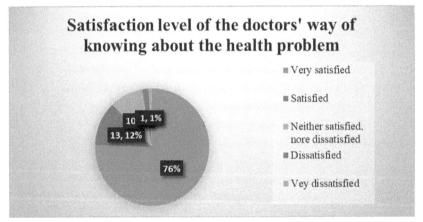

Chart 1. Satisfaction level regarding doctors' skill in knowing about their patients' health

The result indicates that 76% of the patients/their relatives were very satisfied with the way their doctor asks them questions about their health problems. Only 1% of the respondents were dissatisfied with their physicians regarding this question. Thus, the level of dissatisfaction with the doctors' ability to communicate regarding their medical symptoms was extremely low.

Question 2 was also related to the communication skills of the doctor. The participants were asked the following question: How is your doctors' way of giving information and talking to you about your disease? The responses are outlined below:

Statement	Excellent	Good	Average	Poor	Very poor
How is your doctors' way of giving information and talking to you about your disease?	81	10	5	3	1

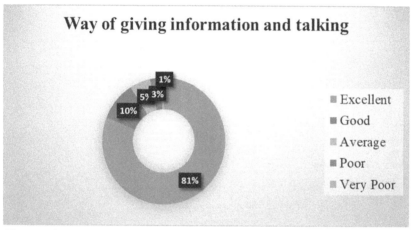

Chart 2. Physicians' way of delivering information/talking to the patient

The results show that the respondents believe that the doctors' ability to converse with their patient is excellent (81%), and 91% of the respondents felt that the doctor's communication skills were either good or excellent. In this way, for this question also, the positive responses from the patients about their doctors were obtained. It is a good indication and the foundation to develop the relationship between the doctors and their patient.

Question 3 regarded the listening skills of the doctor. The researcher asked the respondents how much they agree with the statement that their doctors listened attentively to their problem. The following responses were obtained from the respondents:

Statement	Strongly agree	Agree	Neither agree nor disagree	Disagree	Strongly disagree
My doctor listens to my problems attentively.	77	11	10	1	1

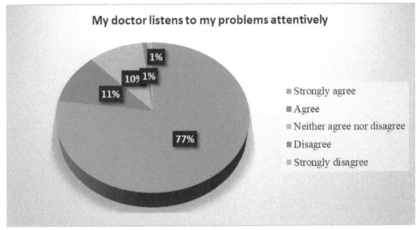

Chart 3. Listening skills of the doctor

The percentage of response is highly in favor of the physicians. About 77% of the respondents expressed a strong liking regarding the listening skills of their doctors.

5.2. Trustworthiness of the Doctor

A virtuous physician needs to be trustworthy. It is a key responsibility of a physician to win trust of the patients because that is a major indicator of their professional success. The first question of this section was, How many days/years have you been receiving treatment from your doctor?

It was a multiple-choice question in which 5 options were given: less than 6 months, 6 months to 1 year, more than 1 year but less than 2 years, more than 2 years but less than 3 years, and more than 3 years. The following responses were obtained:

Acquaintance with the physicians	Value	Percentage
More than 6 months	23	20%
More than 6 months to less than 1 year	21	19.09%
More than 1 year to less than 2 years	26	23.63%
More than 2 years to less than 3 years	24	21.8%
More than 3 years	16	15.48%

This question was important because trust must be developed over a period of time. However, here, we have not considered the frequency of the visits of the patients. Usually, acquaintance with a person can be maintained even in a few visits. It depends upon the approach of the people meeting together.

The next question in this section was asked in the form of a statement in which the respondents had to choose the level of trust-worthiness of their physician. The results are as follows:

Statement	Strongly agree	Agree	Neither agree nor disagree	Disagree	Strongly disagree
My doctor is extremely trustworthy	61	13	09	08	09

About 74% of the respondents expressed agreement with the statement. Nine respondents were neutral on this statement. Seventeen (17) respondents felt that their doctor was not particularly trustworthy. The graphical presentation of the patients' opinion is given below.

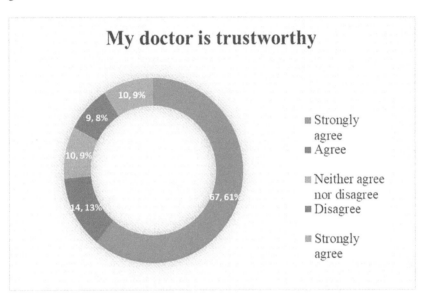

5.3. Transparency of the Physician

The transparency of the physician is of utmost importance for a healthy relationship between doctors and patients. With this in mind, the respondents were asked whether their doctors communicated the effects and side effects of the medications they are prescribing. The respondents had to choose between three options: yes, always; sometimes, if asked; and no, never. Among 110 participants, 39 responded yes, always; 61 responded sometimes, if asked; and 11 responded no, never.

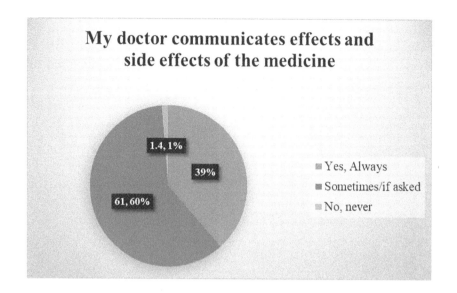

It was the opinion of 61.6% of respondents that their doctors inform them about the effects and side effects of their medicine, but only if they asked for the information. About 39% said that they are always informed about the effects and side effects of the medicines without needing to ask the doctor.

The researcher next asked the respondents about their comfort level with their doctor. The results are as follows:

Statement	Very poor 1	Poor 2	Average 3	Good 4	Excellent 5
My comfort level with my doctor is	00	00	12	34	64

The results show that overall, the comfort level of the patients with their hospital doctor is good or excellent. Moreover, the patients feel that their health-related information will never be disclosed by their physicians (see table below).

	Agree	Disagree
My doctor always maintains confidentiality about my health	107 (97.27%)	03 (2.7%)

5.4. Other Qualities of the Doctor

The researcher tried to measure some other indicators of virtue of the doctors such as their decision-making ability, humanitarian approach, compassion, and discipline. For these qualities, the patients were asked to offer a response on a scale of 1 to 10.

The mean score of each quality has been shown below:

	1	2	3		4	5	6	7	8	9
Decision-making ability								✓		
Humanitarian approach									✓	
Compassion								✓		
Discipline									✓	
Patient-centric approach									✓	

CHAPTER 6

Discussion

This chapter will review the findings presented in the thesis. Findings are derived from three major sources: literature reviews and previous studies, five case studies, and a small survey with hospital patients/ their relatives. The main objective of this research was to analyze medical ethics and its related issues. The discussion topics are divided into three sections according to the three major types of source material listed above. In the first section, the discussion will be conducted on the data procured from the literature review. The findings of the case studies will be discussed in the second section, and in the third section, the researcher will focus on the data procured from the survey.

6.1. Discussion on Literature Review

Medical ethics are viewed as the actions taken by physicians for the welfare and betterment of their patients based on the previous studies and definitions of ethics from different authors. The ethical issues in medical science have been in existence since the ancient times. Medical ethics existed in the ancient civilizations because the medical science in these civilizations was very sophisticated. The more the public holds something accountable, the higher the likelihood that ethics must be followed. The field of medicine is one of the most publicly accountable fields that there is. An individual's life is in the hands of doctor. So negligence or any other unethical practices can be very dangerous for the patients. This thesis reviewed the brutalities and inhumane practices that were performed by officials in the first half of the twentieth century. Deaths (homicides) were quite common for medical experiments. In a 1947 article written by Mellanby, various methods of inhumane medical treatments were described. Sometimes, humans (mostly prisoners and people from concentration camps) were immersed in cold water and died as a result. High-altitude experiments, poison bullet experiments, contagious diseases, and the sterilizations of men and women by x-rays were other human experiments in which live humans were tortured (Mellanby 1947). With a background of these unethical and brutal practices, it was necessary to establish medical ethics codes. In the literature review, the researcher incorporated a graph that chronicles some of the major scandals in medical profession since 1930. These scandals took place before, during, and after World War II. As a result of these scandals, changes/amendments were made to the ethical codes. These scandals included the Syphilis Study, Nazi Experiments, Human Radiation Experiments (1944–1947), the Thalidomide Tragedy (1962), Milgram Study (1963), Gene Transfer Subject Deaths (1999), the Death of Ellen Roche (2001), Nuremberg Code 1947, Kefauver-Harris Amendments 1962, Declaration of Helsinki 1964, *Belmont Report* (1979), HHS/FDA Human Subject Regulations (1981), Common Rules (1981–1991), CIOMS Guidelines (1982), Advisory Committee on Human Radiation Experiments (1994), President's Council on Bioethics (2001), and KGPC (2001).

Medical ethics are based on four major principles—patient autonomy, beneficence, nonmaleficence, and justice—which are found in the Hippocratic oath. These principles and ethical codes were necessary in order to control the unethical practices of the time. As stated by Limentani (1999), ethics codes are the necessary element for the professional control of the behavior of the doctors. Such a long history of incidents of patients' vulnerability has made ethics codes mandatory to ensure a tangible protection to the patients, as well as to the doctors, during challenging circumstances.

From the literature review, it was also observed how ethical decision-making is important for minimizing the cost and maximizing the quality of medical services. It is expected that doctors would adhere to the four fundamental principles of medical ethics. However, some scholars have objected to this view, saying that it is not feasible and practical to adhere to the fundamental principles (autonomy, beneficence, nonmaleficence, and justice) in every circumstance. There are also some ethical theories that have proposed opposite opinions. For example, the utilitarian approach is a consequential approach. It means that if the consequence of the action and decision of the physicians is good and positive, those actions or decisions are moral and ethical. It means that sometimes, the physicians can make a decision that would be beneficial for the patient but the patient has not given consent for that decision. The doctors' decision is ethical because ultimately, the decision is patient centric, and making such decision is therefore ethical. The theory of deontology proposed by Kant is contrary to the viewpoints of utilitarianism. The proponents of the deontology theory state that whatever may be the consequences, the person must adhere to the ethics and codes. The morality thus depends purely upon the action. The simple example in a medical context is that the doctor must tell the truth to the patient and/or their relatives. For example, a patient died after unbearable sufferings in the ICU. The doctor comes out of the ICU and tells the relatives that the patient died peacefully. The intention of the doctor is to give solace and comfort to the patient's relatives that their loved one experienced a calm and peaceful death. According to Kant, in this case, the doctor can be called unethical as he did not tell the truth about the sufferings of the patient. In fact, there is no harm in hiding the truth in this case because the person had already died. But Kant is adamant about the philosophy of truth telling and does not seem to compromise regardless of any circumstances. The deontological approach in decision-making may be appropriate for the individual, but it may not produce a positive outcome to the society (Mandal et al. 2016).

A major viewpoint from the literature review regarding patient autonomy is that although the doctor should respect patients' decisions and patients should be given freedom to make decisions about their health, the doctor can help the patient in making the right decisions. Even though the patient is in a good position (physically and mentally) to make decisions, the decision itself may prove to be wrong in the future. In such a case, the doctors cannot force the patient to change their decision, but the doctors can certainly explain the possible adverse impacts of their decisions. For instance, the patient cannot justify his choice to continue his bad habit of smoking or alcoholism. In such a case, must the doctor respect such an irrational and risky decision of the patient? Ethical dilemmas are everywhere in the medical profession. This has been the focus of the literature review. Medical ethics state that the patient should be given the autonomy to make their own decisions. However, a dilemma exists if the patient is suffering from acute mental and psychological problems: How can they be given the freedom to make decisions regarding their health, especially if it is not good for their health?

It was also observed that cultural issues can bring ethical challenges to the physicians. Some scholars (e.g., see DuVal et al. [2004]) strongly advocate for a requirement for education in ethics and critical thinking to be thoroughly imparted to the doctors so that they can navigate their way through ethical dilemmas.

In the literature review, some of the qualities of a virtuous doctor were discussed. The common qualities proposed by scholars are appropriate decision-making ability, empathetic, high level of emotional quotient, listening skills, and trustworthiness. According to the scholars, a strong doctor-patient relationship can be developed only through the trustworthiness and gentle behavior of the doctor. It was found from the literature review that the relationship between the doctor and the patient is extremely complex; however, it is imperative that this relationship should have a strong foundation of mutual trust as it is the cornerstone of the medical practice.

Being a part of the medical and health-care sector, the pharmacist also has to follow ethical practices. Especially in the context of the medical practitioners, the ethics related to drugs become crucial. The doctor's ethics in the context of pharmaceutical products or drugs are also discussed in the literature review section. It was observed that the pharmaceutical companies promote their products by various unethical means. For example, giving monetary or nonmonetary gifts to the doctors. In such situations, the doctors' ethical obligation is not to succumb to such temptations. It is imperative for the doctor to prescribe the medicines that are cost-effective and safe. This is because not all patients can afford expensive medicines. Moreover, mandatory medicines should never be expensive. As stated by Kamal et al. (2019), one in four patients report that they cannot afford the drugs prescribed by their physicians. The key duties of the medical practitioners observed from the previous studies include ensuring that patients are informed about the drugs, consulting them regarding the necessity of taking drugs, and avoiding bribes in the form of gifts and other benefits from the drug companies as a quid pro quo to promote their products.

The subtopics related to the ethics in the medical sector were discussed with the help of the previous literature. The ethical issues were also observed while analyzing the cases. Hence, in the next section, the discussion on the findings derived from the case studies is conducted.

6.2. Findings and Discussions of Case Studies

The key ethical issues found in the case studies are (1) unjust and discriminatory treatment by the physician, (2) ethical dilemmas arising from religious beliefs/conscience, (3) stressed doctor-patient relationship, and (4) patient autonomy and patient-centric approach. Some unethical practices were also observed with respect to the patient, the commitment level of the doctor, communication problems between the patient and the doctor, pharmacological issues, and surrogacy issues.

In the case studies, it was observed that some doctors were involved in discriminatory practices, especially having made a negative judgment regarding the patient. Discriminatory treatment is never justified, especially when it occurs by a medical practitioner. A doctor's first duty is to be committed to their patients. Lynch (2013) has researched highly publicized cases of doctors who rejected patients on some objectionable grounds such as sexual orientation. In chapter 4, case study 1 described discrimination against the patient (Melissa) based on sexual orientation. This case is supported by Lynch's observation regarding a doctor's mindset to discriminate against their patients. These patients feel offended and insulted due to such treatment from their doctors. The ethical question is whether it is right for the doctor to place his/her religious beliefs above the patient's well-being. If God has not discriminated based on the anatomical structure of the human body, is it ethical for a doctor to discriminate against the patient due to his/her sexual orientation? Sexual orientation is the personal choice of an individual and does not cause harm to other individuals. The doctor's action cannot be justified and cannot be called ethical in any circumstance.

From case study 1, it was determined that the doctor acted irresponsibly. If a doctor cannot continue treatment for any reason, he should explain his decision and recommend another physician. Discontinuing treatment abruptly is an act of extreme irresponsibility.

Case study 2 showed how ethical principles can be followed without any dilemma or conflicts. The doctors in case study 2 demonstrated ethical behaviors such as transparency, patient autonomy, beneficence and nonmaleficence, and a high commitment toward the patient as well as providing decision-making support to the relatives of patients. Every medical professional should follow the responsible and ethical behavior exhibited by the doctors in case study 2. The doctors were an example of how the ethical behavior can be maintained and followed in challenging situations. This case is an ideal case to be included in the education medical students. A sound doctor-patient relationship can only be maintained only through the ethical and responsible behavior of the doctors, who did not leave any chance for conflict or dispute.

Case study 3 was a complicated case in which it was difficult to decide whether the doctors' behavior was right or wrong. On one hand, the doctors' decisions seemed to be ethically correct, yet on other hand, their decision seemed to be ethically incorrect. When disputes or conflicts occur between a patient and their doctor, the patient is equally responsible for the disputes. In case study 3, Maya's thoughts and opinions were irrational as she was ready to sacrifice her life to avoid having a scar on her body. The doctors, concerned for her well-being, performed surgery without her consent. The doctors were successful in following the ethical principles of beneficence and nonmaleficence. But they failed to follow the principle of patient autonomy. In spite of her refusal to consent, the doctors performed the surgery anyway. In such complicated cases, the doctors must listen to their conscience. Quality of life for the patient is the most important detail to protect. If the doctors have to compromise with an ethical principle in order to preserve the quality of life, that action cannot be called unethical. In this case, we can apply the utilitarian theory, which states that if the action/decision has positive outcomes, that action/decision is always ethical. In this case, we also observed a best practice whereby the doctors tried to convince the apprehensive patient to have the surgery by using rational arguments and alternative treatments. This is a good case study for discussing ethical dilemmas in decision-making. It is very difficult to decide whether the action/decision of the doctor was ethical or unethical. Although the doctors' decision to proceed with an unauthorized surgery was the correct choice for the patient's health and safety, they should have tried harder to convince her of its importance.

In case study 4, the ethical actions of the doctors were not involved. Rather, it was a case of surrogacy, one of the disputes that commonly takes place in the medical field. The major finding derived from the case is that yet there is no consensus regarding the ethical position of surrogacy. Though it is a widely discussed topic, no concrete ethical codes have been developed for the act of surrogacy. The laws and ethical codes of surrogacy vary within and among the United States. Outside of the United States, countries have adopted differing viewpoints. Some countries are in favor of surrogacy and the rights of the intended parents, while other countries are against surrogacy and favor the rights of the surrogate mother. Hence, prior to the decision to proceed with surrogacy, the laws and ethics of the country need to be understood. Surrogacy is a desirable practice when the applicable laws are favorable to the intended parents. Otherwise, there is a higher chance of being defrauded by the surrogate mother and bearing a substantial financial and emotional loss. The case also points out that although surrogacy is considered a profession in some states within the United States and in some other countries, the surrogacy contract must recognize that both parties cannot be totally free from emotional upheaval. Hence, everything should be clearly outlined well in advance.

Case study 5 was an excellent example of ethical versus unethical behavior of doctors. The case highlighted the necessary qualities of a virtuous doctor. The case demonstrated that a doctor's job is not just to prescribe medication, but rather the doctor-patient relationship is just as important in the healing process. In this context, patients should always ask themselves questions to determine the type of doctor they would prefer—a doctor who has graduated from a top medical college and shows indifference toward the patient or one who is kind, calm, and compassionate but lacks a prestigious medical degree. Stephen Trzeciak and Anthony Mazzarelli have proven how the compassion of the doctor has an incredible healing power. According to the authors, kindness ensures a healthier life not just for the patients but for the doctors as well. When the doctor delivers an emotional response to his/her patient's ailments, the patient feels that the doctor can actually feel their suffering and has a desire to help the patients relieve their pain. Case study 5 shows how compassion and kindness, along with the doctor's knowledge, can help patients like Meghan recover from her long-standing disease. Dr. Phoebe failed to show compassion and kindness, which ultimately hampered the health and trust of her patient, Meghan. Dr. Smith showed compassion and a desire to help Meghan, allowing him to win the trust of his patient. The following principles were derived from the case study 5:

Do's	Don'ts
Be kind and compassionate to your patient.	Do not prescribe unnecessary dosages of medication.
Know your responsibilities toward your patients.	Do not insult your patient or use any offensive language toward him/her.
Respect your patient	Do not demonstrate aggressive and rude behavior.

Emphasize natural healing and nonpharmacological therapies wherever possible.	Do not ignore your patients intentionally or unintentionally.
Always remember that the patients give you reputation, fame, and wealth.	Do not do anything objectionable which could make your patients feel uncomfortable and embarrassed.

The collective findings from all cases were as follows:

1. In the medical profession, many doctors who are not adequately trained in medical ethics can be discriminatory in their treatment approach and thus violate the ethical principles of justice and equality.
2. In the medical profession, the physicians tend to focus on the life and safety of the patient, which sometimes leads to a compromise of their ethical principles.
3. In order to build a trustworthy relationship with their patients, the virtuous doctor needs to be communicative, compassionate, careful, and cooperative (the four Cs).

6.3. Findings and Discussion on Survey

This chapter will focus on the findings from the primary data. The researcher felt it crucial to communicate with patients and ask them about the behavior and the approach of their treating physicians. Whenever it was not possible to obtain a response from the patient (due to their health issue), the responses were obtained from close relatives of the patient. The findings derived from the survey are discussed below.

The data shows that the doctors' communication with their patients was very clear and unambiguous. The patient could understand the doctor's questions and talk about their health condition because the questions, which were asked by the doctors, were done so in a friendly manner. A positive response was obtained from a majority of the respondents regarding the doctor's manner of asking questions to their patients. The satisfaction level regarding patient communication with their doctors was also relatively high. This confirms a patient-centric approach. Through the question-and-answer session with the patient, the physician should communicate his role as a helper to the patient. Some patients are able to talk about their conditions effectively, while other patients who may be shyer are not able to effectively relate their medical problems. In these cases, the doctor must have the ability to ask appropriate questions from which they can ascertain and diagnose the health issues of the patient.

The survey also showed that the doctors deliver information to the patients in an understandable manner. The research conducted by Kee et al. (2017) focuses on the communication issues between the doctor and the patients. According to the authors, this relationship is extremely complex. Yet it may be the single most important and fundamental component of medical practices. In this communication, many lapses are found, and the authors state that these lapses are often overcome.

According to the survey of American Academy of Orthopaedic Surgeons, 75% of the surgeons believed that their communication with their patients is satisfactory (Kee et al. 2017). However, the same study also found that the patients are not satisfied with the way the doctor communicates with them. In this survey, only 21% of the patients responded that they were satisfied with their communication with the doctors. Kee et al. (2017) evaluated both the verbal and nonverbal communication of the doctors for their survey. Their findings demonstrated that the doctors in their study lacked in showing respect and sympathy for their patients. The study respondents ranked the nonverbal communication skills of their doctors. In the present thesis, the researcher has not differentiated between verbal and nonverbal communication. Rather, the question was regarding communication in general. The elements of communication considered for this research were attentive listening, doctors' skills in understanding the patient's health issues through proper and apt questions, and the doctors' way of delivering information about the patient's illness.

The trustworthiness of the doctors was also measured through the survey responses. As stated by Khullar (2018), trust is vital for the social and economic well-being of the people. However, Khullar

(2018) found that trust is declining in the American society, especially when it comes to trusting doctors. Americans are more skeptical about doctors when the people are from other countries. The author also pointed out that during a recent outbreak of disease, one-third of Americans expressed doubts about the public health officials. According to the respondents, these officials did not share complete, accurate, and trustworthy information to the public. Trust is the cornerstone of any relationship, and in the case of the doctor-patient relationship, it is crucial. The findings derived from our survey were different from Kullar's study. The respondents in our survey demonstrated a high level of trust in their physician. Approximately 79% of the respondents stated that they trust their doctors. In this survey, the period of acquaintance of the patients with their doctors varied; however, the level of trust was high. Maintaining trust is both important and challenging. Once trust is lost, it is difficult to regain. That is why doctors must strive to maintain their trustworthiness and credibility at all times. Trust can only be developed through honesty and transparent communication.

The respondents in the study rated the transparency of their doctors very high. Being transparent in sharing the information is one of the key factors of delivering personalized and sustainable healthcare service according to Henke and Kelsey (2010). There should not be any secrets between the patient and the doctor regarding patient's health and/or illness. The results of our survey show that the patients believed that there is a great amount of transparency between them and their physicians. Of course, this transparency needs to be two-sided. It is the duty of the patients not to hide any health-related issues from their doctors. When the doctors try to conceal medical information, they would be in violation of the ethical principle of patient autonomy. If the doctor is not transparent about the disease, severity, and complexity level, the decision-making process of the patient will be adversely affected. On the other hand, if the doctor is unaware of some medical facts about the patient, the treatment protocol may be compromised or may encounter serious problems. For example, if the patient hides from the doctor that he/she has diabetes, there could be a serious problem with prescribing medicines or during surgery. Of course, nowadays, the doctors obtain all available records (including diabetes, blood pressure) prior to any surgery. But still, it is the responsibility of the patient to be transparent with their physicians.

The survey results also demonstrated a positive response from the patients regarding their comfort level with their doctors. Ranjan et al. (2013) reports that sound communication skills of the physician make the patients comfortable. In the case study of Meghan and her first doctor, Dr. Phoebe, we saw that the approach of Dr. Phoebe was responsible for the breakdown of communication, and Meghan lost her ability to communicate comfortably with the doctor especially when she was insulted for her hearing loss. However, in our survey, we found that the respondents were comfortable when communicating with their doctor. No one rated this question as "very poor" or "poor."

One of the key principles of ethics (though not mentioned in the pillar of medical ethics principles) is maintaining confidentiality, which is perceived as being the patient's right. In the Hippocratic oath, confidentiality is one of the cornerstones of ethical behavior of the doctors. When confidentiality is maintained by physicians, their patients trust them. However, in some circumstances, a breach of confidentiality becomes inevitable. In such cases, the patients should be given information as to why their confidentiality cannot be maintained. The action must have strong reasoning. With this in mind, the respondents of our research were asked whether their doctors maintain confidentiality about their health. A positive response was indicated by 97.21%, whereas only 2.7% of the respondents said that their confidentiality was not maintained.

The respondents gave 8 bands (out of 9 bands) for the humanitarian and patient-centric approach of the doctors and their discipline. They gave 7 bands for the doctors' decision-making abilities and the compassion level of the doctors.

In conclusion, we received an extremely positive response from the participants on all fronts of ethical issues in the clinical settings. We did not observe any conflict, dispute, or feelings of discontent among the patients regarding the medical services being delivered by their doctors.

CHAPTER 7

Conclusion and Recommendations

7.1. Conclusion

The medical profession is highly visible and accountable to the public. As such, it is regulated by a code of ethics. Ethics in medicine has its source in ancient civilizations. Medical ethics, or clinical ethics, aims at delivering sustainable medical services to the patients. A doctor's skills, experience, and competence are important, but along with these core skills, the doctor has to inculcate values and morals. Doctors should always adhere to the four primary principles of ethics: respect for autonomy, beneficence, nonmaleficence, and justice. Apart from that, other virtues that doctors should exhibit are dignity, honesty, commitment, discipline, sound communication, compassion, and sound ethical decision-making. Medical ethics and morals help doctors build trust with patients and establish a good relationship with them.

In the introduction section of this thesis, we discussed the significance of this study on the unethical practices and scandals that are prevalent in the health-care sector. Patients are quite vulnerable to such unethical practices. This research is significant since it sheds light on the various components and factors of medical ethics. The research was designed to investigate the ethical and moral approach of physicians and to analyze the doctor-patient relationship.

We used an analytical and exploratory research approach with an extensive scope. We intentionally kept the topic broad because medical ethics cannot be limited by excluding subtopics such as ethical dilemmas and challenges, doctor-patient relationship, ethical decisions of doctors, etc. So in this analytical study, we covered every possible topic related to medical ethics. The significance of ethics in the clinical setting was analyzed in this thesis. We also focused on situations where doctors have to face ethical dilemmas and potentially may have to compromise one or more ethical principles just to save the life of their patients. We also discussed the conflict between laws and ethics. Doctors face a challenging situation when they have to make a decision during an ethical dilemma.

The topic of medical ethics is widely discussed and researched in the academic circle. Consequently, we were able to conduct extensive research in this area. In the literature review section, *ethics* was defined with the help of definitions from other scholars. The history of bioethics/medical ethics was also reviewed. The focus of the historical review was the twentieth century to the present. We analyzed the unethical and brutal practices of human experimentation that was performed during and after the world wars. The laws and ethical codes became rigid and strict especially in the context of the key principles of ethics. An extensive literature review was undertaken on each ethical principle. Previous studies were reviewed in the context of ethical challenges and dilemmas that doctors have to face. The literature was also reviewed to determine the qualities and virtues of an ideal physician. Ample studies were found, which discussed the doctor-patient relationship. The ethics of prescribing drugs was also discussed in the literature review.

We defined and discussed the research methods that have been used for this thesis. In chapter 3, research methodology, we discussed the research approaches and paradigm. It was confirmed that the present research falls under the paradigm of "social constructivism" and meets all of its criteria. It is a pragmatic research study in which the reality is sometimes ambiguous (especially during ethical dilemmas). For this research, data was collected from primary and secondary sources as well. Along with a literature review, a case study analysis and a survey were conducted to have concrete and substantial data that is required for the research. The problem complexity was discussed, and the pluralistic domain of interest and values was confirmed. The analysis of case studies was the major method used; hence, it was important to know what the case study analysis is and its crucial role in qualitative research. For the case study research, we considered five different cases. Along with the case studies, we also conducted a survey of patients or/and their relatives and analyzed these methods of collecting data. The approach used for the case study analysis was a multiple-embedded case study method. The parameters of selecting the cases were described. We explained the survey method that was used to collect the primary data. The research methodology section reviewed the questions included in the questionnaire by explaining their types. The researcher is also obligated to adhere to ethics principles, which are explained in the same chapter.

In chapter 4, case study analysis, we explained the steps that were followed for the analysis of the cases. The first case highlighted the discriminatory approach of a doctor after realizing that his patient was homosexual. We discussed the case on the parameters of medical ethics. The second case highlighted the ethical practices of the doctors in the case of an elderly woman whose condition was critical. This was an ideal case to make the students familiar with the ethical principles that should be followed in challenging situations and thus avoid disputes. The third case was based on the violation of the first principle of ethics—patient autonomy. In this case, the doctors performed surgery on a young woman without her consent. It was a lifesaving operation. Instead of patient autonomy, the doctors followed the paternalistic approach. The patient filed a lawsuit against the doctors and the hospital. The fourth case focused on surrogacy and the ethical issues related to surrogacy. This case shed light on the debate over surrogacy and how the laws of each state of the United States as well as other countries are different regarding surrogacy. In case five, two opposite experiences of a patient were examined, and a comparative analysis was conducted to analyze the ethical and unethical approaches used by the two doctors treating the patient.

Chapter 5 analyzed a small survey conducted with the patients and/or their relatives regarding their satisfaction with their physician. The physicians received extremely positive responses from all 110 respondents. Based on this extensive study, we would like to suggest some recommendations for the future studies.

7.2. Recommendations

It is highly recommended that the similar studies should be conducted in other parts of the world. Sometimes, cultural and social factors also have an impact on ethical issues though the fundamental issues are similar everywhere.

1. There are several topics that were not included in this study on which case study analysis is essential. With this in mind, future researchers are encouraged to analyze cases relating to other issues such as euthanasia, unethical practices in the drug industry, suicide cases, and other such topics.
2. We conducted a small survey in with 110 respondents. Future research should be conducted using a wider scope and a larger number of respondents.
3. This research can be a longitudinal research project since the scope of the topic is extensive.
4. We only used the survey method for collecting primary data. A qualitative analysis could be conducted through semistructured and unstructured interviews in which patient opinions can be related in detail.
5. Our survey was conducted using only patients and/or their relatives. Therefore, we cannot comment on the perspectives of the medical practitioners. It is highly advisable that future interviews/surveys should be conducted with the doctors as well.
6. It is recommended that research in medical ethics should be conducted on regular basis.

CHAPTER 8

Ethics Consultation Curriculum

This work was done when I did my practicum (at a hospital) under the supervision of Dr. Amy Van Dyke. I am so grateful to her for the opportunity she gave me to do this work. This chapter is about ethics consultation curriculum. It is designed for ethics consultants at hospital settings to guide patients to make appropriate decisions. It is a curriculum designed to teach medical students, bioethics students, chaplains or postgraduate researchers, and physicians and any other professionals who want to be part of the ethics consultation. Three cases have been reviewed which will be the focus of the cases which is taught. For instance, it is primarily a case about:

- Informed consent
- End-of-life decision-making
- Advance directive interpretation

These cases have been simplified to focus on the issues described above. The primary role for role-playing is the teaching focus. This includes a list of items you want the participants to highlight in the role-play, such as the following:

- Did they follow the best practices guidelines in American Society for Bioethics and Humanities (ASBH) book?

- o   Introduction of self, role, goals, format of meeting, rules surrounding what to expect, etc.
- Did the consultant show/use/incorporate knowledge of Ohio Revised Code in the consult?
- General secular bioethics principles (respect for autonomy, beneficence, nonmaleficence, and justice).
- Ethical and Religious Directives for Catholic Health Care Services (ERDs).

The participants have been scored. Scoring tool has been used to determine how well the consultant did their job.

Case Preparation

Case 1
Surrogate Decision-Making

Medical Background

This case concerns an 89-year-old widow, Mrs. Sarah Lahue, who presents with delirium, schizoaffective disorder, and dementia. The patient is disoriented and uncooperative. She is mostly nonverbal. Her judgment is impaired due to her inability to grasp and analyze information and come to an appropriate decision. She is currently unable to make decisions regarding her health care.

The patient has had a diagnosis of mental disorder for over 20 years. Her medications had been stabilizing her mental condition; however, in the past year, she has been becoming confused and agitated in spite of her medication. Attempts were made to change her medications during a previous hospital stay for her deteriorating mental condition. She did experience some improvement on the new medication. However, her two sons, who have power of attorney, opposed the medication change and returned her to her prior medication. The patient also has a history of a CVA, coronary artery disease, hypertension, decubitus ulcer, and esophagitis.

Psychosocial Information

Ms. Lahue is an 89-year-old widow whose husband died 5 or 6 years ago. She has two sons (who are the surrogate decision-makers) and two sisters. She has been living with one of her sons prior to admission to the hospital. She has an eighth grade education.

Reason for the Ethics Consult

The ethics consultation was requested by Mrs. Laue's physician, Dr. Guy Cho, to assist in decision-making regarding her treatment.

113

There is disagreement between the physician and the patient's two sons regarding the continuation of her current drug protocol, which is having side effects and is believed to be contributing to her deterioration. During a previous mental hospitalization, Dr. Sugar Kurup attempted to change her medication, but her son "sabotaged" the treatment, insisting that she stay on the old medication.

Stakeholders Present for the Ethics Consult

- Physician—requested the consult after a disagreement with the patient's sons concerning treatment.
- Ethics consultant—facilitate the meeting to ensure that all parties (the sons and the physician) have an opportunity to express their views regarding the patient's treatment.
- Two sons—surrogate decision-makers, representing the patient, and making decisions on her behalf.

Surrogate Decision-Making

Surrogate decision-making is common in health-care settings where the patient cannot make sound decisions due to their health conditions. In these instances, the patient requires the presence of a surrogate decision-maker—an individual who will act in the best interests of the patient by taking into account the personal values, goals, and wishes of the patient.

This paper will analyze a case study of a patient undergoing medical treatment for a mental illness and cardiovascular issues. Due to her mental status, a surrogate has been assigned to make medical decisions on her behalf. The paper discusses aspects of general bioethics principles and laws and analyzes whether the participants in the case adhered to those principles and to the American Society for Bioethics and Humanities (ASBH) guidelines for health-care ethics. As a Catholic health-care institution, the Ethical and Religious Directives for Catholic Health Care (ERDs) will be analyzed.

Case Study and Participants

In this case, the patient, Mrs. Sarah Lahue, is an elderly woman with a 20-year history of mental illness. She presents with delirium, schizoaffective disorder, and dementia. Additionally, the patient has cardiovascular disease. A psychiatric consultation was ordered that revealed that the patient was confused, uncooperative, and mostly nonverbal. Therefore, she would not be able to make informed personal/medical decisions.

Psychological disorders can have an impact on one's ability to make decisions. In the case of delirium, it is associated with a substantial disturbance in one's mental abilities leading to reduced awareness of the environment and confused thinking. Hence, rather than have the patient make decisions, the ethics consultant needs to engage an external third party to make decisions on her behalf. The ethic consultant's engagement of a surrogate decision-maker is justified as the information provided further suggests that the patient is uncooperative, confused, and mostly nonverbal. Even when she talks, she is verbally aggressive. Since she cannot communicate clearly due to her health condition, her sons (who are the surrogate decision-makers) take on the role of surrogate decision-maker. The sons have been providing critical information to the ethics consultant especially regarding the history of her health conditions and where she has received treatment.

Mrs. Lahue has been on Stelazine and other drugs that have worked well for over 20 years; however, a closer examination suggests that those drugs are no longer effective. As a result, the patient may have to use different drugs that are proven to be more effective in treating her condition. The decision to continue using or to discontinue using the previous drugs is a matter that must be decided with the input from the patient's surrogate decision-makers. The psychiatric consultant's expert opinion is that the drugs must be changed because the old medication has negative side effects, which may be the cause of her confusion and stiffness. In addition to the current consultant's opinion, the referring physician, Dr. Cho, had also suggested the need to start using the new drug and abandon the old medicine. While the consultant's and Dr. Cho's advice was focused on the patient's health and safety, the surrogate decision-makers were of a different opinion. They rejected the recommendations of the physicians even after being informed that the old medication is likely the cause of the patient's delirium.

Primary Roles for Role-Playing

In this case study, the primary roles for role-playing includes the following:

- Patient
- Patient's guardians (son 1 and son 2)
- First ethics consultant
- Second consultant

Critical Items in the Role-Play

a. Strict adherence of the guidelines issued in American Society for Bioethics and Humanities (ASBH) books (ASBH, n.d.). This includes using appropriate communication skills, being empathic to the patient, and allowing the stakeholders to share their sorrow, emotions, and anger.

b. Demonstrate effective application of the Ohio Revised Code (Section 2133.08). Consent to treatment may be given by the appropriate individual(s) in accordance with the following descending order of priority:
   - ✓ The guardian of the patient, if any
   - ✓ The patient's spouse
   - ✓ An adult child of the patient or, if there is more than one adult child, a majority of the patient's adult children who are available within a reasonable period of time for the consultation with the patient's physician
   - ✓ The patient's parent
   - ✓ An adult sibling of the patient or, if there is more than one adult, a majority of the patient's adult sib-

lings who are available within a reasonable period of time for that consultation

✓ Or the nearest adult who is related to the patient by blood or adoption and who is available within a reasonable period of time for that consultation

c. Demonstrate effective application of the principles of bio-ethics such as respect for autonomy, justice, beneficence, and nonmaleficence.

d. Demonstrate ERDs:

✓ Promote human dignity.

✓ Promote mutual respect to the patient and the two sons, who are the surrogate decision-makers.

✓ Serve patient and her family with respect.

✓ Provide a full range of religious and spiritual care for the patient and her family.

Scoring Participants

The case study contained four active participants: the psychiatric consultant (Dr. Kurup), the patient's physician (Dr. Cho), and the patient's two sons. The tables below have been used to rank the ethicist. An overall score of 1–10 is regarded as "poor," a score of 11–20 is "good," while a score of 21–30 reflects "excellent."

Table 1. Ethics consultant

Participant: Ethics consultant	Total possible score = 30
Assessment/analysis skills • Was ethics question formulated correctly? (5 points) • Review of relevant ethics literature, policies, standards, and laws (3 points) • Were appropriate individuals involved in consultation? (3 points) • Communication with patient, POA, surrogate, medical professionals, etc.—both written and verbal (3 points)	

Process skills
  1. Facilitation skills including ensuring effective communication between parties and ensuring all parties are heard (5 points)
  2. Educate regarding ethics policies/laws	

Interpersonal skills (3 points)
  1. Communication skills including ability to listen, show respect, support, and empathy (5 points)
  2. Ability to identify and respond to barriers to communication (3 points)	

References

ASBH. 2011. *Core Competencies for Healthcare Ethics Consultation* 2nd Edition.

Beachamp, et al. 2013. *Principles of Biomedical Ethics* 7th Edition. New York: Oxford University Press.

LAWriter. n.d. "Chapter 4731: Physicians; Limited Practitioners." Retrieved from http://codes.ohio.gov/orc/4731.

United States Conference of Catholic Bishops. 2018. *Ethical and Religious Directives for Catholic Health Care Services* 6th Edition.

Case 2
End-of-Life Decision-Making

Medical Background

This is a case concerning end-of-life care for a 45-year-old, Mr. Benjamin Friedman, who was diagnosed with nonresectable colon cancer and is in the end stages of his life. On admission to the hospital (from the nursing home) for sepsis, the patient was unable to move or communicate. He was on a ventilator and on dialysis. The patient had little chance of survival. He was given antibiotics and steroids for the treatment of the sepsis. Because of his situation, aggressive vasopressor therapy was started to offset his dropping blood pressure. Regardless of the treatment, his pressure continued to range between 30 and 40 systolic on maximum vasopressor therapy. Within 24 hours, he had become anuria, developed massive generalized edema, and was oozing fluid from her skin.

Psychosocial Information

No information is given concerning Mr. Friedman's educational background. Only scanty information has been provided about his family. We know that he has only one daughter, Janet, who is 23 years old and the surrogate decision-maker by ORC hierarchy.

Reason for the Ethics Consult

The ethics consultation was requested by Dr. Mary Cummins, the patient's physician. There was disagreement between her and the patient's daughter, Janet, regarding his end-of-life care. Dr. Adu-Tutu believed that there were no other treatment options for Mr. Friedman—that all treatment options had been exhausted and he was not responding. However, the patient's daughter, the surrogate, was not ready to allow the physician to stop treatment. She wanted all procedures taken to prolong the life of her father.

Stakeholders Present for the Ethics Consult

- Physician—requested the consult
- Ethics consultant—the facilitator of the meeting
- Janet—the patient's daughter who was the surrogate decision-maker

End-of-Life care Decision-Making

End-of-life decision-making is a growing need in many hospitals and nursing homes, especially in the ICU. It can be overwhelming to be asked to make health-care decisions for someone who is dying and is no longer able to make his/her own decisions. It is even more difficult if you do not have written or verbal guidance. How do you decide what type of treatment is right for the patient? Even when there are written documents, some decisions still might not be clear since the documents may not address every situation that could occur.

This case focuses on end-of-life decision-making. It involves a case study of a patient who is terminally ill and cannot make decisions for himself. Its main focus is to determine whether the participants in the case are able to make appropriate decisions for the patient. It examines elements that the surrogate decision-maker needs to consider when making a decision on behalf of the patient. It will also look at using relevant laws, the Ethical and Religious Directives for Catholic Health Care (ERDs), and general principles of bioethics.

Case Study and Relevant Knowledge

This is a case of end-of-life care, which involves a 45-year-old man, Mr. Friedman, who was diagnosed with nonresectable colon cancer and is in the end stages of his life. On admission to the hospital (from the nursing home) for sepsis, the patient was unable to move or communicate. He was on a ventilator and on dialysis. The patient had little chance of survival. He was given antibiotics and steroids for the treatment of the sepsis. Because of his situation, aggressive vaso-pressor therapy was started to offset her dropping blood pressure. Regardless of the treatment, his pressure continued to range between 30 and 40 systolic on maximum vasopressor therapy. Within 24 hours, she had become anuria, developed massive generalized edema, and was oozing fluid from his skin.

The Physician and the Family (Jane)

Indeed, the situation was difficult to navigate. The physician, Dr. Adu Addai, thought that treatment could no longer continue. Mr. Friedman had no advance directive to guide the physician or his daughter. When there is no advance directive, the physician's first challenge is to determine who to approach about critical care deci-sions. In this case, the patient's daughter was the surrogate and was not ready to stop treatment. She wanted all procedures taken to pro-long the life of her father. In order to arrive at decisions that are appropriate to the situation, all concerned need to share a common appreciation of the patient's condition and prognosis.

Early in the discussion, it is important to determine the accu-racy of the family's (Janet's) knowledge and the degree of accep-tance of the patient's condition and prognosis. It is useful to have Janet describe her expectations for what will happen medically with the patient in the future. If the family's appreciation of the clinical situation differs significantly from the physician's, it is usually not possible to achieve an appropriate plan of care at that time. In the event that the family cannot provide direction, the physician should state clearly the default position (cardiopulmonary resuscitation) and agree to meet with the family again after initiating efforts to bridge the lack of common ground using additional tests and consultations with experts and involving the ethics committee, social workers, the chaplain, and other resources.

The Consultant: Ethicist (Ethics Committee)

Indeed, the medical information the physician shared with Mr. Friedman's daughter created a huge burden for her. No one wants to receive such information about their parent and their eventual death. The ethics consultant needs to express words of empathy with the patient and the daughter. A central, although not exclusive, focus of ethics consultant is to facilitate the consultation. He/she focuses on several issues: who requested the consult, why was it requested, what service the ethics consultants can provide, and the patient's likely outcome. The ethics consultant must make sure that Janet feels comfortable, listened to, and not confused.

In making her decision, the ethics consultant must know that some states like have enacted legislation that clearly defines the hierarchy of decision-makers, and the state law will direct the decisions when they exist. Without legal guidance, the most common hierarchy is the spouse, then the adult children, and then the parents. The ethics consultant, in consultation with the physician and the family, should encourage decisions that best incorporate the patient's values, realizing that the most appropriate source for this information may not be the next of kin. The ethics consultant should be prepared to provide emotional support when family members verbally express, for the first time, the expectation of their loved one's impending death.

Approaches to End-of-Life Care Decision-Making

In deciding about end-of-life care, two approaches are used. The first approach is to put yourself in the place of the person who is dying and try to choose as he or she would choose. This is called "substitute judgment." Some experts believe that decisions should be based on substitute judgment whenever possible. The second approach, known as "best interest," is to decide what would be best for the dying person. This is sometimes combined with substitute judgment.

Since Janet is making the decision on behalf of her father, the ethics consultant and the physician should guide her to think about the following questions:

- Has her father ever talked about what he would want at the end of life?
- Has her father expressed an opinion about how someone else was being treated?
- What were her father's values in life? What gave meaning to life? Maybe it was being close to family—watching them grow and making memories together. Perhaps just being alive was the most important thing.

In consultation with the ethics consultant, if the patient's daughter, Janet, like her father, insists to have "everything be done" and no headway can be made, the ethics consultant should allow Janet a few days to go home, sit down, and reflect about the medical facts and other information given to her by the physician. She needs time to process the information to help her make a thorough decision without any coercion or influence. A follow-up meeting involving the social worker, the chaplain, and the physician should be arranged to help her with the decision.

Primary Roles for Role-Playing

The primary roles for role-playing in this case study include the following:

- Patient
- Jane, patient's daughter
- Physician
- Ethics consultant

Items in the Role-Play

1. ASBH book *Core Competencies for Healthcare Ethics Consultation* must be strictly followed. Appropriate communication skills must be used—the ethics committee must listen carefully and empathically to the moral distress experienced by all the parties involved. All participants must be given time to communicate effectively and be heard by other participants by sharing their views and asking questions. Opportunities should be given to the physician to provide the necessary medical information the daughter needs to make a decision. The daughter should then be allowed to express how she understands her father's medical situation. Clarification should be made about the medical facts where appropriate—relevant medical facts should be elicited where the need arises. The ethics consultant should actively listen and maintain eye contact. The committee members should maintain a distraction-free environment to provide a professional consultation.

2. Demonstrate effective application of the Ohio Revised Code (ORC).

3. Demonstrate effective application of the principles of bioethics such as autonomy, justice, beneficence, and nonmaleficence.

4. Demonstrate the Ethical and Religious Directives for Catholic Health Care Services (ERDs). Catholic health care is committed to the care of the whole person—body, mind, and spirit. We listen, we explain, and we serve with compassion. Treatment embraces the physical, psychological, social, and spiritual dimensions of the human person.

Scoring Participants

The case study contained three active participants: the patient's physician (Dr. Adu Addai), the ethicist, and the patient's daughter

(Janet). The tables below have been used to rank the ethicist. A score of 1–10 is regarded as "poor," a score of 11–20 is good, while a score of 21–30 reflects "excellent."

Table 1. Ethics consultant

Participant: Ethics consultant	Total possible score = 30
Assessment/analysis skills • Was ethics question(s) formulated correctly? (5 points) • Review of relevant ethics literature, policies, standards, and laws (3 points) • Were appropriate individuals involved in consultation? (3 points) • Communication with patient, surrogate, medical professionals, etc.—both written and verbal (3 points)	
Process skills 1. Facilitation skills including ensuring effective communication between parties and ensuring all parties are heard (5 points) 2. Educate regarding ethics policies/laws (3 points)	
Interpersonal skills 1. Communication skills including ability to listen, show respect, support, and empathy (5 points) 2. Ability to identify and respond to barriers to communication (3 points)	

References

ASBH. 2011. *Core Competencies for Healthcare Ethics Consultation* 2nd Edition.

Beachamp et al. 2013. *Principles of Biomedical Ethics* 7th Edition. New York: Oxford University Press.

LAWriter. n.d. "Chapter 4731: Physicians; Limited Practitioners." Retrieved from http://codes.ohio.gov/orc/4731.

United States Conference of Catholic Bishops. 2018. *Ethical and Religious Directives for Catholic Health Care Services* 6th Edition.

Case 3
Advance Directive

Medical Background

This case involves a 67-year-old woman, Ms. Gloria Opoku Agyemang, who has been in the ICU for over 21 days. She has had previous admissions to the ICU. From a medical perspective, the patient requires hemodialysis, is on a trach vent with a high level of oxygen needed, and has a bacterial infection. Ms. Agyemang has had several strokes in the past; however, her neurological functioning is reported to be somewhat more stable now than it had been previously. Since being admitted on this occasion, the patient has not had adequate decision-making capacity.

Psychosocial Information

Ms. Agyemang has three adult children—Asantewaa, Boatemaa, and Adoma—who are considered to be the appropriate decision-makers for the patient. There was no information available regarding her educational background.

Reason Given for the Ethics Consult

Ms. Agyemang does not have an advance directive and is unable to make informed decisions for her own care. The ethical issue in this case is to determine who is the appropriate decision-maker for the patient. It is believed that the family is acting the best interest of the patient.

Ethics Consultant Present for the Consult

- Physician—requested the consult
- Ethics consultant—facilitator
- The three adult children—according to ACT 169, are the appropriate decision-makers for the patient

Advance Directive Interpretation

When a person is unable to make key decisions regarding his/her life due to their health conditions, medical personnel first look to see if the patient has an advance directive for their care. An advance directive is defined as a document by which a person makes a provision for health-care decisions in case he/she is unable to make such decisions in the future (Patient Rights Council, n.d.). There are several types of advance directives. This case involves a review specifically focusing on the issue of the patient's advance directive and makes suggestions of what the participants ought to highlight in the role-play. Finally, the scoring of the participants will be provided.

Review of the Case Study

In this case, Ms. Gloria Opoku Agyemang is a patient who has had multiple admissions to the ICU. Presently, she has been in the ICU for more than 20 days. Patients who remain in the ICU for an extended period of time will need various medical interventions. Unfortunately, Ms. Agyemang lacks the capacity to make decisions about her health care. Her physician, Dr. Sahai, can provide medical intervention; however, he has to adhere to the recommendations of the ethics consultation. While an advance directive would normally provide the needed information for how to intervene, there is none in this instance. Ms. Nata has three adult children, who, by law, are permitted to make decisions on her behalf. Unfortunately, the children are generally unreachable. Even when they can be reached, they are reluctant to cooperate and cannot reach consensus about their mother's care. The lack of consensus among the children and their unavailability make it difficult to provide medical intervention in a timely manner to save the life of the patient.

Comment About the Case

This case is a perfect example of where a bioethics consultation is needed and should be followed. The consultation process itself is very important. The consultant should focus on two things: (1) attempting to gather information and (2) developing a good relationship with the adult children. The consultant should follow a standardized process and create an atmosphere of respect with the adult children. The reasons for respecting the views of the adult children include the following:

1. Promote the value of the patient
2. Facilitate the acceptance and implementation of a resolution
3. Clarify options that are ethically valid
4. Encourage learning

In this case, communication is key. The family members need to gain a common viewpoint on the decisions to be made in the best interest of the patient.

Primary Roles for Role-Playing

In this case study, the primary roles for role-playing include the following:

- Patient (Ms. Agyemang)
- Ethics consultant
- Doctor (Dr. Sahai)
- Three adult children (Asantewaa, Boatemaa, and Adoma)

Items to be Highlighted in the Role-Play

The manner in which the consultant handles the case should meet the best practices as described in American Society for Bioethics and Humanities (ASBH) guidelines. For instance, the consultant should use the appropriate communication skills to help the children to dialogue, improve their relationships, and build trust so that they could make better decisions. Again, the consultant must follow the ASBH guidelines by approaching the children so that they could make a decision on behalf of their mother. Additionally, recording and keeping notes regarding children's reluctance was is important in this case.

In seeking a solution to the problem, three key items that need to be emphasized in the role-play are (1) communication coaching, (2) clarification of policy, and (3) mediation. Communication coaching involves the consultant communicating with the adult children to build trust to improve their relationship and will result in enhanced united decision-making. For a productive discussion to occur, the children should understand the patient's prognosis and the potential benefits, as well as the consequences of each treatment alternative. To help the children make their decision, the consultants should clarify the hospital's policy regarding the challenge the patient is facing. This may include policies about triage at the ICU. Mediation is another strategy that the consultant should employ to minimize conflict or divergent opinions among the children. The children should be brought together to reach consensus in an ethical manner. Even when consensus seems impossible, the consultant should help the children to dialogue. Dialogue not only improves shared decision-making but also builds trust.

The ERDs encourage and respect advance directives, respect choices of surrogate decision-makers, honor patients' right to make treatment decisions, and respect decisions to forgo treatment, the distinction between ordinary or proportionate means (morally obligatory), and extraordinary or disproportionate means (morally optional). Catholic health care has the responsibility to treat those in need in a way that respects the human dignity and eternal destiny of all. Since a Catholic health-care institution is a community of healing and compassion, care is not limited to the physical; it also embraces the psychological, social, and spiritual dimensions of the person.

Scoring Participants

The case study contained five active participants: the patient's physician (Dr. Sahai), the ethicist, and the patient's three children. The tables below have been used to rank the ethicist. A score of 1–10 is regarded as "poor," a score of 11–20 is "good," while a score of 21–30 reflects "excellent."

Table 1. Ethics consultant

Participant: Ethics consultant	Total possible score = 30
Assessment/analysis skills • Was ethics question formulated correctly? • Review of relevant ethics literature, policies, standards, and laws • Were appropriate individuals involved in consultation? • Communication with patient, POA, surrogate, medical professionals, etc.—both written and verbal	
Process skills 1. Facilitation skills including ensuring effective communication between parties, ensure all parties are heard 2. Educate regarding ethics policies/laws	
Interpersonal Skills 1. Communication skills including ability to listen, show respect, support, empathy 2. Ability to identify and respond to barriers to communication	

References

ASBH. 2013. *Core Competencies for Healthcare Ethics Consultation* 2nd Edition.

Beachamp et al. 2013. *Principles of Biomedical Ethics* 7th Edition. New York: Oxford University Press.

LAWriter. n.d. "Chapter 4731: Physicians; Limited practitioners." Retrieved from http://codes.ohio.gov/orc/4731.

Stanford. (n.d.). *What Are the Basic Principles of Medical Ethics?* Retrieved from https://web.stanford.edu/class/siw198q/web-sites/reprotech/New%20Ways%20of%20Making%20Babies/EthicVoc.htm.

REFERENCES

AbuAbah, F., A. Alwan, Y. Al Jahdali, et al. 2019. "Common Medical Ethical Issues Faced by Healthcare Professionals in KSA." *Journal of Taibah University Medical Science* 14 (5): 412–417.

Adolphus, M. n.d. "How to Undertake Case Study Research." *Emerald Publishing*. Retrieved from https://www.emeraldgrouppublishing.com/research/guides/methods/case_study.htm?part=1.

Alkabba, A., G. Hussain, A. Albar, A. Bahnassy, and M. Qadi. 2012. "The Major Medical Ethical Challenges Facing the Public and Healthcare Providers in Saudi Arabia." *Journal of Family and Community Medicine* 19 (1): 1–6.

Bain, L. 2018. "Revisiting the Need for Virtue in Medical Practice: A Reflection Upon the Teaching of Edmund Pallegrino." *Philosophy, Ethics, and Humanities in Medicine* 13 (4). https://doi.org/10.1186/s13010-018-0057-0.

Beauchamp, G. 1998. "General Surgeon and Clinical Ethics: A Survey." *Canadian Journal of Surgery* 41 (6): 451–454.

Beauchamp, T., and J. Childress. 2001. *Principles of Biomedical Ethics*. New York: Oxford University Press.

Braveman, P., S. Kumanyika, J. Fielding, et al. 2011. "Health Disparities and Health Equity: The Issue Is Justice." *American Journal of Public Health* 101 (1): 5149–5155.

Buchanan, A. E., and D. W. Brock. 1990. *Deciding for Others: The Ethics of Surrogate Decision Making*. New York: Cambridge University Press.

Cayton, H. 2005. "Some Thoughts on Medical Professionalism and Regulations." *Defining and Developing Professionalism Conference*. Association for the Study of Medical Association.

Chaix-Couturier, C., I. Durand-Zaleski, D. Jolly, and P. Durieux. 2000. "Effects of Financial Incentives on Medical Practice: Results from a Systematic Review of the Literature and Methodological Issues." *International Journal for Quality in Health Care* 12: 133–142.

Chandra, S. 2017. "Trust and Communication in a Doctor-Patient Relationship: A Literature Review." *Journal of Healthcare Communication* 3 (36): 1–6.

Charles, C., A. Gafni, and T. Whelan. 1999. "Decision Making in the Physician-Patient Encounter: Revisiting the Shared Treatment Decision-Making Model." *Social Science and Medicine* 49: 651–661.

Chipidza, F., R. Wallwork, and T. Stern. 2015. "Impact of the Doctor-Patient Relationship." *The Primary Care Companion for CNS Disorders* 17 (5). doi:10.4088/PCC.15f01840.

Churchill, L. 1999. "Are We Professionals? A Critical Look at the Social Role of Bioethics." *Daedalus* 128 (4): 253–274.

Colotla, I. 2003. *Operation and Performance of International Manufacturing Networks, PhD Thesis.* Cambridge, UK: Cambridge University.

Crowe, S., K. Cresswell, A. Robertson, et al. 2011. "The Case Study Approach." *BMC Medical Research Methodology* 11 (100). https://doi.org/10.1186/1471-2288-11-100.

Dempski, K. M. 2009. "Informed Consent." In *Nursing Law and Ethics*, edited by S. J. Westrick and K. Dempski, 77–83. Sudbury, MA: Jones and Bartlett.

Drescher, J. 2002. "Ethical Issues in Treating Gay and Lesbian Patients." *Psychiatric Clinics of North America* 25 (3): 605–621. doi:10.1016/S0193-953X(02)00004-7.

DuVal, G., B. Clarridge, G. Gensler, and M. Danis. 2004. "A National Survey of U.S. Internists' Experience with Ethical Dilemmas and Ethics Consultation." *Journal of General Internal Medicine* 19 (3): 251–258. doi:10.1111/j.1525-1497.2004.21238.x.

Dworkin, G. 1988. *The Theory and Practice of Autonomy.* New York: Cambridge University Press.

Easterby-Smith, M., R. Thorpe, and A. Lowe. 2002. *Management Research: An Introduction*. London: SAGE Publications.

Evan, J. 2016. "The Changing Ethics of Health Care." *Caring for the Ages*. Retrieved from https://www.caringfortheages.com/article/S1526-4114(16)30143-3/pdf.

Farber, H. J., A. M. Capra, J. A. Finkelstein, P. Lozano, C. P. Quesenberry, N. G. Jensvold, F. W. Chi, and T. A. Lieu. 2003. "Misunderstanding of Asthma Controller Medications: Association with Nonadherence." *Journal of Asthma* 40 (1): 17–25.

Figar, N., and B. Dordevic. 2016. "Managing Ethical Dilemma." *Economic Themes* 54 (3): 345–362.

Gibbon, M., C. Limoges, H. Nowotny, S. Schwartzman, P. Scott, and M. Trow. 1995. *The New Production of Knowledge: The Dynamics of Science and Research in Contemporary Society*. London, Thousand Oaks, and New Delhi: SAGE Publications.

Henke, N., and T. Kelsey. 2011. "Transparency: The Most Powerful Driver of Health Care Improvement?" *McKinsey & Company*. Retrieved from https://www.mckinsey.com/~/media/mckinsey/dotcom/client_service/Healthcare%20Systems%20and%20Services/Health%20International/Issue%2011%20new%20PDFs/HI11_64%20Transparency_noprint.ashx.

Hinduism. 2013. "Medical Ethics." *Hinduism Today*. Retrieved from https://www.hinduismtoday.com/modules/smartsection/item.php?itemid=5340.

Jochen, V., and R. Winau. 1999. "Informed Consent in Human Experimentation Before the Nuremberg Code." *BMJ British Medical Journal* 313 (7070): 1445–1449.

Jones, J. W., L. B. McCullough, and B. W. Richman. 2005. "Truth-Telling About Terminal Disease." *Surgery*. 137 (3): 380–382. doi:10.1016/j.surg.2004.09.013.

Kamal, R., C. Cox, and D. McDermott. 2019. "What Are the Recent and Forecasted Trends in Prescription Drug Spending?" *Peterson-Kaiser Health System Tracker*. Retrieved from https://www.healthsystemtracker.org/chart-collection/recent-forecasted-trends-prescription-drug-spending/#item-start.

Kant. 1964. *The Doctrine of Virtue*. New York: Harper and Roe.

Kee, J., H. Khoo, I. Lim, and M. Koh. 2017. "Communication Skills in Patient-Doctor Interactions: Learning from Patient Complaints." *Health Professional Education* 4(2): 97–106.

Kidder, Rushworth. 2003. *How Good People Make Tough Choices: Resolving the Dilemmas of Ethical Living*, 63. New York: Harper Collins. ISBN 0-688-17590-2.

Kim, W. 2012. "Institutional Review Board (IRB) and Ethical Issues in Clinical Research." *Korean Journal of Anesthesiology* 62 (1): 3–12.

Kullar, D. 2018. "Do You Trust Medical Profession? *New York Times*. Retrieved from nytimes.com/2018/01/23/upshot/do-you-trust-the-medical-profession.html.

Mandal, J., D. Ponnambath, and S. Parija. 2017. "Bioethics: A Brief Review." *Tropical Parasitology*, 7 (1): 5–7.

Jones J. W., L. B. McCullough, and B. W. Richman. 2005. "Truth-Telling About Terminal Disease." *Surgery.* 137 (3): 380–382. doi:10.1016/j.surg.2004.09.013.

Masel E. K., A. Kitta, P. Huber, T. Rumpold, M. Unseld, S. Schur, et al. 2016. "What Makes a Good Palliative Care Physician? A Qualitative Study About the Patient's Expectations and Needs When Being Admitted to a Palliative Care Unit." *PLoS One* 11 (7).

Mishra N. N., T. Bhatia, N. Kumar, V. L. Nimgaonkar, L. S. Parker, and S. N. Deshpande. 2014. "Knowledge and Attitudes of Mental Health Professionals Regarding Psychiatric Research." *Indian J Med Res.* 139 (2): 246–51.

Nandi, P. 2000. "Ethical Aspects of Clinical Practices." *Arch Surg* 135 (1): 22–25. doi:10.1001/archsurg.135.1.22.

Nowotny, H., P. Scott, and M. Gibbons. 2003. "Introduction: 'Mode 2' Revisited: The New Production of Knowledge." *Special Issue: Reflections on the New Production of Knowledge* 41 (3): 179–194. https://www.jstor.org/stable/41821245.

Pellegrino E. 2002. "Professionalism, Profession, and the Virtues of the Good Physician." *Mt Sinai J Med.* 69 (6): 378–384.

Pennings, G. 2012. "Ethical Issues in Infertility Treatment." *Best Practice & Research Clinical Obstetrics Gynaecology* 26 (6): 853–863.

Prioresch, P. 1997. "The Hippocratic Oath, Abortion, Greek Homosexuality, and the Courts." *Hacienda Publishing*. Retrieved from https://haciendapublishing.com/medicalsentinel/ hippocratic-oath-abortion-greek-homosexuality-and-courts.

Prokopijevic, M. 1990. "Surrogate Motherhood." *Journal of Applied Philosophy* 7 (2): 169–181.

Pugmire, D. 1978. "Altruism and Ethics." *American Philosophical Quarterly* 15 (1): 75–80.

Raina, R., P. Singh, A. Chaturvedi, H. Thakur, and D. Parihar. 2014. "Emerging Ethical Perspective in Physician-Patient Relationship." *Journal of Clinical and Diagnostic Research* 8 (11): XI01–XI04.

Ranjan, P., Archana Kumari, and A. Chakrawarty. 2015. "How Can Doctors Improve Their Communication Skills?" *Journal of Clinical and Diagnostic Research* 9 (3). doi:10.7860/ JCDR/2015/12072.5712.

Rasmussen, L. B. 2011. *Interactive Leadership: Paradigms and Models.* Lyngby, DK: DTU Press.

Rich, K. 2020. "Introduction to Bioethics Decision Making." In *Nursing Ethics*, edited by J. Butts and K. Rich. Burlington: Jones and Bartlett Learning.

Rushworth, K. 2003. *How Good People Make Tough Choices: Resolving the Dilemmas of Ethical Living.* New York: Harper Collins.

Salloch, S. 2016. "Same Same but Different: Why We Should Care About the Distinction Between Professionalism and Ethics." *BMC Medical Ethics* 17 (44). doi:10.1186/s12910-016-0128-y.

Saniotis, A. 2007. "Changing Ethics in Medical Practice: A Thai Perspective." *Indian Journal of Medical Ethics* 4 (1): 24–25. doi:10.20529/IJME.2007.008.

Satterwhite, W. M., R. C. Satterwite, and C. E. Enarson. 1998. "Medical Students' Perception of Unethical Conduct at One Medical School." *Academic Medicine: Journal of the Association of American Medical Colleges* 75 (5): 529–531.

Saxena, P., A. Mishra, and S. Malik. 2012. "Surrogacy: Ethical and Legal Issues." *Indian Journal of Community Medicine*, 37 (4): 211–213. doi: 10.4103/0970-0218.103466.

Schloendorff v. Society of New York Hospital, 211 N.Y. 125 2020.

Singh, J., and M. Ivory. 2015. "Beneficence/Nonmaleficence." In *The Encyclopedia of Clinical Psychology* edited by R. Cautin and S. Lilienfeld. Wiley Blackwell.

Shelton W. 1999. "Can Virtue Be Taught?" *Acad Med* 74 (6): 671–674.

Shrivastava, S., P. Shrivastava, and J. Ramasamy. 2014. "Exploring the Dimensions of the Doctor-Patient Relationship in Clinical Practice in Hospital Settings." *International Journal of Health Policy Management* 2 (4): 159–160.

Simons, H. 2009. *Case Study Research in Practice.* London: SAGE.

Sjetne, I., O. Bjetnaes, R. Olsen, H. Iversen, and G. Bukholm. 2011. "The Generic Short Patient Experiences Questionnaire (GS-PEQ): Identification of Core Items from a Survey in Norway." *BMC Health Services Research* 11 (88): 1–11.

Stavropoulou, C. 2012. "The Doctor-Patient Relationship: A Review of the Theory and Policy Implications." In *The LSE Companion to Health Policy*. Cheltenham: Edward Elgar Publishing Limited. ISBN 9781781004234.

Sturman, A. 1997. "Case Study Methods." In *Educational Research, Methodology and Measurement: An International Handbook* 2nd Ed. edited by J. P. Keeves, 61–66. Oxford: Pergamon.

Swindell, J., A. McGuire, and S. Halpern. 2010. "Beneficent Persuasion: Techniques and Ethical Guidelines to Improve Patient's Decisions." *Annals of Family Medicine* 8 (3).

Thomas, G. 2011. "A Typology for the Case Study in Social Science Following a Review of Definition, Discourse and Structure." *Qualitative Inquiry* 17 (6): 511–521.

Varelius, J. 2006. "The Value of Autonomy in Medical Ethics." *Medicine, Health Care and Philosophy* 9 (3): 377–388. doi:10.1007/s11019-006-9000-z.

Vaz, M. and K. Srinivasan. "Ethical Challenges and Dilemmas for Medical Health Professionals Doing Psychiatric Research." *Indian Journal of Medical Research* 139 (2): 191–193.

Wamock, M. 1985. *Question of Life: The Warnock Report on Human Fertilisation and Embryology.* Oxford and New York: Basil Blackwell.

What Is Bioethics? n.d. *Center for Ethics and Humanities in the Life Sciences. College of Human Medicines. Michigan University.* Retrieved from https://bioethics.msu.edu/what-is-bioethics

Whitehouse, P. 2003. "The Rebirth of Bioethics: Extending the Original Formulations of Van Rensselaer Potter." *American Journal of Bioethics* 3: 26–31.

Yadav, H., R. Jegasothy, S. Ramkrishnappa, J. Mohanjraj, and P. Sena. 2019. "Unethical Behaviour and Professionalism Among Medical Students in a Private Medical University of Malaysia." *BMC Medical Education* 19 (218). https://doi.org/10.1186/s12909-019-1662-3.

Yousef, R. 2017. "Awareness, Knowledge and Attitude Toward Informed Consent Among Doctors in Two Different Cultures in Asia: A Cross-Sectional Comparative Study in Malaysia and Kashmir, India." *Singapore Medical Journal* 48 (6): 559–565.

Zokefli, Y. 2018. "The Ethics of Truth Telling in Health-Care Settings." *The Malaysian Journal of Medical Sciences* 25 (3): 135–139.

Zubovic, D. 2018. "Ethical Dilemmas of Nurses and Physicians in the Primary Health Care Setting." *Hospice and Palliative Medicine International Journal* 2 (5): 280–284.

Zukauskas, P., J. Vveinhardt, and R. Andriukaitiene. 2018. "Philosophy and Paradigm of Scientific Research." In *Management Culture and Corporate Social Responsibility.* IntechOpen. https://dx.doi.org/10.5772/intechopen.70628.

APPENDIX

Questions and Answers: Bioethics

Features of the American System of Federalism, the System's Advantages and Disadvantages for Issues of Bioethics, and a Current Bioethics Debate Where Federalism Has Important Implications

US federalism is a system of dual sovereignty between the two levels of governments: federal and state. The power of the federal government is shared among the executive, the legislature, and the judiciary (Fossett). Although the national government is sometimes presumed to have overridden powers at the expense of state governments, the fact is that both systems are interdependent (i.e., they are mutually dependent upon one another). The system of governance creates a division of power both among the branches of government and between the levels of government, which prevents the ratification of laws and policies that may be contrary to the will of the people. Finally, this system of governance purposefully averts the formation of a tyrannical government.

The US Constitution specifically outlines the responsibilities of each level of government, thereby ensuring a balance of power. This system of government lends itself to inclusivity, allowing the interests of various parties, from the local to the national level and whether majority or minority, to be taken into consideration. This division of power between the federal and the state governments both allows and encourages citizens to become more involved in government policies and lawmaking.

Several bioethical issues will test the effectiveness of the balance of power within the US system of governance. One such issue is that of "designer" babies (i.e., babies that are genetically engineered in vitro to ensure the presence or absence of particular genes or characteristics). Scientists have begun to enumerate the advantages associated with genetically altered fetuses. These advantages include protection from diseases such as Alzheimer's and Down's syndrome, protection against inherited medical conditions such as diabetes, and an increase in life expectancy (Fordham 1475). However, this technology could pose potential threats to its users because it has not yet been proven to be 100% safe. For instance, the procedure is relatively new and is not error-free and could cause harm or termination of the fetus. If the government is expected to protect its citizens from potential harms, it is likely that both the national and state governments will develop laws around this issue to regulate procedures and ensure safety.

The US system of federalism can also be associated with disadvantages related to bioethics issues. For instance, federalism allows states and national governments to act independently; bioethics regulations enacted at separate levels can conflict. For instance, the national government may legalize designer babies for factors such as protection of people against diseases, yet a state might enact laws prohibiting the practice based on discrimination against individuals who cannot afford the expensive procedure. Thus, it may be that the procedure will only be legal in a few states while other states may ban the practice, ultimately leaving the decision on legality to be made in the courts.

The Ethical Principles Upon Which Surrogates Make Decisions on Behalf of Incapacitated Patients and Challenges Encountered by Surrogates in Such Instances

The well-being of incapacitated patients depends on decisions made by others on issues such as their medical treatment, other health-related issues, and finances at the end of their life. Given that incapacitated patients are unable to make their own health-care decisions, surrogate decision-makers are appointed to make decisions for them. There are certain inherent factors that affect the accuracy of the surrogate's decision, such as their own personal risk attitudes, choices, and personality (Kaplunov and Harvey). For example, a doctor or a patient's relative might choose to withdraw life support from a patient, but that might not be the will of the patient if he/she was in a position to make that decision. Consequently, there are principles that control the actions of surrogate decision-makers regarding the well-being of incapacitated patients. These principles include (1) deciding the best interest of the patient and (2) the need to understand the patient's preferences and values before making a decision (Pope). The ethical principle of beneficence—the need to do good, be kind, be helpful, and be generous—also controls the decisions made by a surrogate decision-maker.

Despite the ethical principles that guide the decisions of the surrogate, there remain some unresolved challenges. These challenges include and may be impacted by the degree of relationship between a surrogate decision-maker and the beneficiary (i.e., the incapacitated patient) or how well the surrogate decision-maker(s) know the patient. Herein lays the challenge of choosing a surrogate. When a condition requires the need for a hasty decision, there may not be time to choose a surrogate who is a close family member and would know the patient's preferences and wishes. Instead, a physician might be required to take that role despite not knowing the patient well. Failure to determine the preferences of the beneficiary and instead acting on their own preferences may lead to making an impulsive or incorrect decision (Kaplunov and Harvey). The failure to consult courts and hospital ethics boards may also lead to making an impulsive decision. The nationality of the surrogate may also affect the decision made. Research has found that in Britain, the closer the biological relationship, the more likely that an impulsive decision will be made (Kaplunov, 266). However, among Europeans, a close biological relationship will yield a more accurate decision.

Why the End-of-Life Decision-Making Is a Challenge and What Can Be Done to Make It More Manageable and Satisfying

End-of-life decision-making can be a challenging issue because the patient is unable to make decisions for himself. Instead, a third party must balance what they believe is "best" for the patient against what is "best" according to the medical professionals. The treatment plan as well as the patient outcome might be quite different between the two factions. When the surrogate decision-maker and the care team have opposing views on the care protocol, a potentially futile dispute occurs (Tejwani et al.). As Tejwani et al. denote, this happens most often when the surrogate decision-maker is a close family member of the patient. Unlike the care team that bases their decision on the potential health outcome of the patient, surrogate decision-makers who are family members tend to make their decision based on personal interest, emotions, and their feelings toward the patient. There are laws recognizing advance directives or "living wills" that allow individuals to communicate their end-of-life wishes to their family, friends, and health-care professionals while they are still healthy. Unfortunately, few people actually formalize an advance directive, and thus, an accurate decision based on the wishes of the patient is often not made.

Issues around end-of-life decision-making can be addressed through the proper implementation of the 1990 Patient Self-Determination Act. The act outlines individuals' rights to make decisions regarding their end-of-life care and ensures that patients certify the advance directive by communicating their wishes to others, especially health-care institutions. A 2008 report found that while about 92% of Americans were aware of the availability of an advance directive, only about 36% had adopted one (Tejwani et al.). Increasing the percentage of individuals with an advance directive would decrease the chances of an individual's end-of-life wishes being ignored. That goal can be achieved by requiring beneficiaries of Medicare and Medicaid to communicate their end-of-life wishes and values and identifying their surrogate decision-makers.

Creating a collaboration of surrogates, including family members, the medical care team, and the hospital ethics committee, may also enhance the chances of the patient's wishes being honored although it could also lead to multiple disagreements. In the event that the patient has not stated their preferred surrogate, states such as Texas have given the medical care team the right to make the final decision based on the best interest of the patient. This approach might also resolve the challenges of disagreement among appointed surrogates.

Comparing and Contrasting the Physician/Patient Relationship with the Researcher/Subject Relationship, How They Have evolved, and the Ethical Challenges They Share

The physician/patient relationship can be traced back to ancient times with Egypt involving "the clergy representing the patients to the gods, which was within a medical practice based on magic and mysticism" (Osorio 400). During the fifth century BC, the physician/patient relationship was improved to address issues such as natural changes that could impact individual health. The "disease model" was adopted at the beginning of the eighteenth century AD and considered patients to rank above physicians. This change enhanced the physician/patient relationship because the needs of the patient were now dealt with as individual problems requiring the physician to experience the illness through the eyes of the patient. The physician/patient relationship was also enhanced by the rapid rise of hospitals in the 1700s, which led to less-privileged patients having access to care and, consequently, physicians interacting more frequently with previously passive patients (Osorio, 401).

Contrast this with the researcher/subject relationship in which the experience of a research subject was less considered. This impacted the relationship in meaningful ways such as whether the relationship between the researcher and the subject involves financial gain were less considered. The specifics of the relationship between a researcher and the subject were less considered in research. But currently, those factors are more considered and are central in research studies.

A strong and healthy relationship, be it the physician/patient relationship or researcher/subject relationship, improves the outcomes of clinical activities and research outcomes because the involved parties collaborate toward the same motive: to create knowledge (Stavropoulou). In both the relationships, there are possible ethical challenges such as the following:

> Lack of informed consent of the subjects and the patients. This includes (a) involving a subject in research and/or a medical intervention without their consent and (b) failing to inform research subjects and patients of the risks that may be involved in study participation.

> Sharing private information about the subjects and patients involved.

In contrast, the researcher/subject relationship often involves offering a stipend for participation in the study. The physician/patient relationship, however, does not permit stipends to be offered to a physician for services offered to the patient. Although all parties involved in both relationships benefit from the collaboration, the patients directly benefit from a relationship with a physician because it enhances health-care service outcomes. Subjects in a research study do not benefit directly from the results of a study. The researcher/subject relationship is precipitated by the researcher recruiting the subjects for the study and may involve personal and/or professional friends. But in the case of physician/patient research, the physician does not choose the patient from personal or professional friends, and the study has more of an institutional culture.

The Role of Informed Consent in Bioethics, What Shaped the Development of Informed Consent in Bioethics, the Reason for Its Continued Importance in this Field, and the Differences Between the Way Informed Consent Developed in the Clinical Setting Compared to the Research Setting

The concept of informed consent in bioethics is important because medical interventions require patient understanding and acceptance, particularly with care that may be associated with potential ethical issues. Consequently, informed consent of the person involved (particularly a patient) ensures that there is communication with the patient before a medical intervention can be undertaken so that they can choose whether to accept or decline the medical intervention (Sorta-Bilajac, 89). The choice of a medical operation is based on the patient having been informed and understands the benefits, harms, and risks associated with various medical alternatives. Essentially, when there is good and open communication between the patient and the physician, the patient-physician relationship is enhanced, thus fostering trust. Informed consent also reduces the potential of ethical issues. In the case where an ethical problem arises after a medical intervention, it is easier to resolve the case since the intervention was undertaken with the consent of the patient, thus valuing the principle of respect for autonomy, which ensures "an attempt to instill relevant understanding, to avoid forms of manipulation, and to respect persons' right" (Beauchamp and Childress, 121).

Fundamentally, the concept of informed consent in bioethics was not a central topic before the 1970s. But technological advancements leading to advances in medical practice and the development of bioethics and ethical human subject research were central in the integration of the concept of informed consent in the field of bioethics. Those changes created ethical issues due to research and medical intervention abuses, and therefore, the need for informed consent in bioethics arose. For instance, in a 1947 case, the Nuremberg Medical Tribunal found that sixteen people were guilty of medical research abuse (Presidential Commission for the Study of Bioethical Issues, 7). The result of the tribunal was the adoption of the Nuremberg Code that emphasized the need for informed consent during research. There is also the Tuskegee Syphilis Study from 1932 to 1972 where the participants in the study did not provide informed consent. These extreme abuses marked need for the adoption of various clauses, including the Declaration of Helsinki and the National Commission, which stressed the need for informed consent in bioethics. Notably, there are no specific differences that were exhibited in the development of the concept of informed consent in clinical practices and the research setting. That is because as medical abuses in both clinical and research settings increased, various bodies, policies, and regulations were passed to stress the need for informed consent in medical interventions and research. As medical research, technological advancements, and medical intervention advances continue, ethical issues will continue to arise, and the need for new parameters around the concept of informed consent will be needed to reduce potential ethical issues.

Bioethics as a Profession or Not and the Movement to Certify Ethics Consultants and Draft Code of Ethics by the American Society for Bioethics and Humanities (ASBH)

Various factors are considered when determining whether an occupation should qualify as a profession. Hence, when an occupation falls short of the necessary features, the professionalization of the occupation might be undesirable. The field of bioethics has some characteristics that can arguably make it be considered a profession. Among those attributes is the fact that since the 1980s, medical schools in the United States are increasingly including courses in bioethics as part of the curriculum. However, there are also some characteristics that make it undesirable to consider bioethics a profession. Notably, bioethics has begun to be a requirement for professional accreditation in various health-care professions, including nursing. Therefore, bioethics could be defined as an integral part of health-care programs that are considered professions rather than a single profession itself where a physician can engage in professional activities such as teaching physiology but, at the same time, engaging in bioethics activities (Klugman, 6). Bioethics does not have the social and economic power of other health-care professions where the need to avoid research and clinical practice abuses becomes the primary area of concern. While bioethics requires its professionals to excel in their field, bioethicists do not necessarily receive payment for their services. Conversely, there are cases where the majority of a person's salary may be derived from bioethics activities, factors that positively impact the argument for bioethics to be considered a profession.

The American Society for Bioethics and Humanities (ASBH) is a body that has tried to address the issue of whether or not bioethics is a profession. The ASBH has taken steps to certify ethics consultants, and in 2018, 138 individuals completed the certification examination. Only two applicants were not certified to be health-care consultants (Siegler). The need to certify ethics consultants introduces the issue of jurisdiction and supports the view of bioethics as a profession (Klugman, 11). That is because a profession usually receives oversight through jurisdictional regulations. The issue of whether or not bioethics should be considered a profession impacts the decision to have a code of ethics for the profession, given that codes of ethics act as an axis on which a profession can evolve. In 2005, a proposal was made to the ASBH to include a code of ethics for ethics consultants. A survey following the proposal showed that 61% of the respondents supported a code of ethics for bioethics (Tarzian et al., 4). Accordingly, a recommendation for the same was made to the ASBH.

Factors Contributing to Moral Distress for Clinicians, Why It Persists, and What Can Be Done to Address It

Clinicians, like other medical professionals, may encounter challenges associated with doing what is ethically correct according to their personal viewpoint versus what is required by institution policies and practices. This situation is referred to as moral distress. These challenges are not limited to the medical profession but rather persist widely throughout the gamut of professions. Factors that contribute to moral distress include personal values, qualities and experiences, the culture, and the world's view/perception of events. Personal qualities that may contribute to moral distress include role perception by a clinician is defined as the confidence of a clinician regarding his/her own skills and competencies (Burston and Tuckett, 4). This factor may be exacerbated by the clinician's level of authority. Clinicians may also be impacted by their expectation of standards of care, which influenced the worldview versus what that individual considers to be ethical.

Ethical dilemmas are some factors that can lead to moral distress, given that institutional, personal, and ethical decisions often tend to conflict. There are, for instance, circumstances where a nurse may have to follow an institutional protocol or the specific instructions of a physician despite understanding that taking such an action is not ethically ideal. Accordingly, the nurse/physician relationship can impact moral distress for a nurse through poor understanding and/or lack of collaboration contributing to the level of moral distress. Additional institutional factors that can contribute to moral distress include staffing levels, resourcing (which includes, but is not limited to, time and finances), and other site-specific factors (Burston and Tuckett, 5). Inadequate resourcing can lead to an inability to provide a high level of health care, which heightens moral distress through the knowledge that more could have been done if adequate resources had been allocated.

Moral distress can be reduced if the risk factors contributing to the distress can be accounted for and addressed. Actions such as adequate staffing and appropriate resourcing in the health-care institution, emphasizing and enhancing an interprofessional relationship, adopting flexible institutional protocols, and culture will go far in reducing moral distress. In addition, ethics education can help to develop personal qualities and broaden the worldview of clinicians. Implementing these actions would help to ensure that a health professional would not have to face an ethical dilemma just because the institution's protocol, culture, or superiors dictate that a certain action be taken.

The Principle "Action Is Not Based on Information Alone" and a Case to Affirm That Principle

Information is necessary for action, but according to a key principle of the ethical practice of public health, "action is not based on information alone" (Petrini). In many instances, a precautionary action is taken when all of the required information is not available. Conversely, one may have all the information required to take action but fail to take any action. In these cases, an individual's values regarding the policies, fundamental values, and dignity are substituted instead and override the correct decision. Even when all information is readily available, subjective values are used in interpreting the information and taking action.

In 2015, a family from the United States adopted several children from a nation where the prevalence of tuberculosis (TB) is high. After the children arrived in the United States, a screening was completed to determine the health of the children. They were found to be infected with TB; however, the disease was inactive and the children were not contagious. Immigration health officials advised the family to seek medical attention for the health condition and explained the potential risks that are associated with not immunizing the children or following a treatment protocol should a child develop TB symptoms (Ortmann). The religious beliefs of the adoptive parents prevented them from immunizing the children; hence, the children were never treated or immunized against TB.

Later, one of the children exhibited TB symptoms. The family waited several months before taking the child to the hospital. When they finally decided to visit a pediatrician, the child was diagnosed with multidrug-resistant TB (MDR-TB) symptoms. A health-care professional visited the family to provide services in the home following the directly observed treatment protocol (DOT) practiced in the United States (Ortmann). The parents refused to allow treatment because it was a violation of parental and privacy rights, given that the nurse had visited the family's home. In this case, the parents had information on the risks involved if they failed to immunize their children and were instructed to consult a physician if the children exhibited TB symptoms. However, their value system caused them to ignore symptoms and refuse treatment despite having information about the appropriate actions to take.

WORKS CITED

Beauchamp, Tom L., and James F. Childress. 2013 *Principles of Biomedical Ethics* 7th Ed. New York: Oxford University Press.

Burston, Adam S., and Anthony G. Tuckett. 2013 "Moral Distress in Nursing: Contributing Factors, Outcomes, and Interventions." *Nursing Ethics* 20.3: 312–324.

Doyle, Cavan. 2019. "Biomedical Ethics and Law Class Lectures."

Eckenwiler, Lisa A., et al., eds. 2007. *The Ethics of Bioethics: Mapping the Moral Landscape.* Baltimore: The Johns Hopkins University Press.

Fordham, Brigham A. 2011. "Disability and Designer Babies." *Valparaiso University Law Review* 45.4: 159–21

Fossett, James W., et al. 2007. "States and Moral Pluralism." *Hastings Center Report* 37.6: 24–35

Kaplunov, Elizabeth, and Nigel Harvey. 2017. "Incapacitated Patients' Wellbeing: Surrogate Decision Making." *III International Scientific Symposium on Lifelong Wellbeing in the World (Wellso 2016)*, vol. 19. Future Academy. doi:10.15405/ epsbs.2017.01.36.

Kayhan, Parsi. 2019. "History of Medicine and Bioethics Class Lectures."

Klugman, Craig M. 2008. "Is Bioethics a Profession?" *Online Journal of Health Ethics* 5.2: 6

Ortmann, Leonard W., et al. 2016. "Public Health Ethics: Global Cases, Practice, and Context." *Public Health Ethics: Cases Spanning the Globe*, 3–35. Cham: Springer.

Osorio, José Henry. 2011. "Evolution and Changes in the Physician-Patient Relationship." *Colombia Medica* 42.3: 400–406.

Petrini, Carlo. 2010. "Theoretical Models and Operational Frameworks in Public Health Ethics." *International Journal of Environmental Research and Public Health* 7.1: 189–202. doi:10.3390/ijerph7010189.

Pope, Thaddeus Mason. 2012. "Legal Fundamentals of Surrogate Decision Making." *Chest* 141.4: 1074–1081. doi:10.1378/chest.11-2336.

Presidential Commission for the Study of Bioethical Issues. 2016. "Informed Consent Background." https://bioethicsarchive.georgetown.edu/pcsbi/sites/default/files/1%20Informed%20Consent%20Background%209.30.16.pdf.

Siegler, Mark. 2019. "The ASBH Approach to Certify Clinical Ethics Consultants Is Both Premature and Inadequate." *The Journal of Clinical Ethics* 30.2: 109–116.

Sorta-Bilajac, Iva. 2016. "Informed Consent in UNESCO Bioethics Documents." *Hrestomatija Hrvatskoga Medicinskog Prava.* Pravni fakultet Sveučilišta u Zagrebu-Biblioteka Udžbenici.

Stavropoulou. 2012. "The Doctor-Patient Relationship: A Review of the Theory and Policy Implications." In *The LSE Companion to Health Policy*, 314–326. Cheltenham: Edward Elgar Publishing Limited. ISBN 9781781004234.

Tarzian, Anita J., Lucia D. Wocial, and ASBH Clinical Ethics Consultation Affairs Committee. 2015. "A Code of Ethics for Health Care Ethics Consultants: Journey to the Present and Implications for the Field." *The American Journal of Bioethics* 15.5: 38–51.

Tejwani, Vickram, et al. 2013. "Issues Surrounding End-of-Life Decision-Making." *Patient Preference and Adherence* 7: 771. doi:10.2147/PPA.S48135.

ABOUT THE AUTHOR

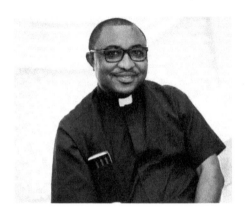

Rev. Fr. Dr. Emmanuel Adu Addai, born in Maase-Offinso, Ghana, and ordained in 2009, is a priest of the Catholic Archdiocese of Kumasi, Ghana. He acquired Masters in Bioethics and Licentiate in Moral theology at Boston College, Massachusetts, and the doctorate in bioethics at Loyola University Chicago Stritch School of Medicine, United States. He has taught as high school tutor and served as chaplain. He has some publications to his credit: "African Women/Girls and HIV/AIDs: The Issue of Justice", "Pawa Series: A Comprehensive Guide to Christian Religious Studies For Senior High Schools and co-authored "A Wonder Personality and his Journey of Faith: Biography of Archbishop Sarpong". He is currently working as parochial vicar at St. Paul's Church, Westerville, Ohio, and in charge of the Ghanaian Catholic Community at St. Anthony, Columbus, Ohio, United States.

CPSIA information can be obtained
at www.ICGtesting.com
Printed in the USA
JSHW052250030521
14283JS00007B/22